T0211099

Bipolar Disorder
in Young People

Bipolar Disorder in Young People

A Psychological Intervention Manual

Dr. Craig A. Macneil

Dr. Melissa K. Hasty

Dr. Philippe Conus

Professor Michael Berk

Professor Jan Scott

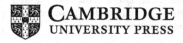

CAMBRIDGE
UNIVERSITY PRESS

University Printing House, Cambridge CB2 8BS, United Kingdom

One Liberty Plaza, 20th Floor, New York, NY 10006, USA

477 Williamstown Road, Port Melbourne, VIC 3207, Australia

4843/24, 2nd Floor, Ansari Road, Daryaganj, Delhi - 110002, India

79 Anson Road, #06-04/06, Singapore 079906

Cambridge University Press is part of the University of Cambridge.

It furthers the University's mission by disseminating knowledge in the pursuit of education, learning and research at the highest international levels of excellence.

www.cambridge.org
Information on this title: www.cambridge.org/9780521719360

First published 2009

A catalogue record for this publication is available from the British Library

Library of Congress Cataloging in Publication data
Bipolar disorder in young people : a psychological intervention manual / edited by Craig A. Macneil ... [et al.].
    p. ; cm.
    Includes bibliographical references and index.
    ISBN 978-0-521-71936-0 (pbk.)
1. Manic-depressive illness in adolescence.   2. Manic-depressive illness–Treatment.   3. Cognitive therapy.   I. Macneil, Craig A.
II. Title.
    [DNLM: 1. Bipolar Disorder–psychology.   2. Adolescent.   3. Bipolar Disorder–therapy.   4. Cognitive Therapy–methods.   WM 207 B616 2009]
    RC516.B5224 2009
    616.89'5–dc22

                                                                    2008044206

ISBN 978-0-521-71936-0 Paperback

....

Every effort has been made in preparing this book to provide accurate and up-to-date information which is in accord with accepted standards and practice at the time of publication. Although case histories are drawn from actual cases, every effort has been made to disguise the identities of the individuals involved. Nevertheless, the authors, editors and publishers can make no warranties that the information contained herein is totally free from error, not least because clinical standards are constantly changing through research and regulation. The authors, editors and publishers therefore disclaim all liability for direct or consequential damages resulting from the use of material contained in this book. Readers are strongly advised to pay careful attention to information provided by the manufacturer of any drugs or equipment that they plan to use.

Contents

Preface

Bipolar disorder can have a significant effect on adolescent development and has traditionally been associated with poor outcomes, both symptomatically and in terms of psychosocial functioning.

There is growing evidence for the effectiveness of psychological interventions for bipolar disorder, particularly individual and family-based cognitive behavioral therapy (CBT). Furthermore, there is emerging evidence that both psychological and pharmacological interventions may be more effective early in the course of the disorder. However, there is currently very little literature describing the unique challenges and opportunities relating to psychological work with a young bipolar population, and there are currently no published clinician manuals relating to this population.

This is the first book to describe a manualized psychological intervention for people in adolescence and early adulthood who are experiencing bipolar disorder. It was developed by clinicians working in a specialist bipolar team at the Early Psychosis Prevention and Intervention Centre (EPPIC) in Melbourne, Australia, in collaboration with Professor Jan Scott, an eminent researcher in the field of bipolar disorder. EPPIC is a leading clinical and research center for young people experiencing mental health difficulties, and this manual was developed from clinical experience and research evidence gathered by the bipolar team over the past five years.

The manual describes specific issues affecting a young bipolar population and offers clinicians advice on how to manage challenges such as difficulties in engagement, comorbidity, family issues, and developmental factors which impact on the person's adaptation to the disorder. In addition to providing a review of the relevant current literature, it has a strong focus on practical interventions that have proven effective when working with this population. This is illustrated through numerous "real world" case studies, and text boxes describing tips and techniques for the clinician.

This manual describes eight modules addressing key areas commonly experienced when working with this population (assessment and engagement, psychoeducation and adaptation, medication adherence, targeted cognitive behavioral interventions, social rhythm regulation, family work, comorbid issues, and relapse prevention). These can be drawn from separately, or combined as part of formulation-based intervention. As some aspects of the intervention are likely to be important whether a cognitive behavioral or other therapeutic model is followed, we have not "labeled" all the introductory chapters as specifically "cognitive therapy." However, we do provide a chapter that highlights specific cognitive behavioral techniques that we have found to be particularly useful in working with adolescents and young adults.

As with any psychological intervention, previous training and experience are highly advisable, and good clinical supervision is strongly recommended. Specifically, experience of working with young people, experience of providing cognitive behavioral and family interventions, in addition to experience of working with people with bipolar disorder, will allow a clinician to obtain the best outcomes from this manual. The range and depth of necessary skills cross disciplinary boundaries, so this book represents a collaboration between individuals who use a multi-faceted psychobiosocial approach to helping young people confronted by the challenge of coping with bipolar disorder.

Acknowledgements

The authors would like to thank a number of people who have contributed to the development of this manual.

Thanks to Professor Pat McGorry and the ORYGEN Research Centre for their support.

Many thanks also to Professor Andrew Gumley, Dr. David Miklowitz, Dr. Jeffrey Young, Dr. Christine Padesky, Dr. William Miller, Dr. Peter Hayward, Professor David Fowler, Dr. Ellen Davies-Edwards, Dr. Melanie Fennell, Dr. Leanne Hides, Ms. Lisa Henry, and Mr. Kingsley Crisp for permission to cite their work, or for their comments on drafts of the manual.

Thanks to the staff at Cambridge University Press, particularly B.K., Laura Wood, Richard Marley, and Annie Lovett for all their help in the development of the book, Dave Edwards for copy-editing, and also the staff at the Royal Melbourne Hospital Library for their work in obtaining a significant number of the journal articles referred to in the manual.

Special thanks to the dedicated and dynamic staff at EPPIC in Melbourne, and to the young people attending the service who gave us permission to use their stories or their artwork, particularly E. B., S. M., M. K., J. F., S. F., V. N., S. V., D. R., A. F., Y. H., and N. R. We also want to thank these young people for teaching us about bipolar disorder.

This manual is dedicated to our partners and families.

Introduction

Background to the manual

In recent years there has been growing recognition of the importance of psychological therapies for people with bipolar disorder (Scott & Colom, 2005). While biological and genetic factors appear to play a significant part in the etiology of the disorder (Pekkarinen et al., 1995; Hyman, 1999; Berrettini, 2000), and medication, particularly mood stabilizers, remains the first line of treatment for many clinicians, pharmacological interventions are not universally effective. Numerous reviews have found that even lithium – considered by many to be the "gold standard" of mood stabilizers – is effective in preventing relapse of symptoms for only 32–6% of people with bipolar disorder at 2-year follow-up (Prien et al., 1984; Gelenberg et al., 1989; Silverstone et al., 1998), with up to 87% of people relapsing at 5 years despite good medication adherence (Keller et al., 1993).

The heterogeneity of people with bipolar disorder, its psychosocial impact, and the complexity of the disorder itself led the US National Institute of Mental Health to conclude: "It is clear that pharmacotherapy alone does not meet the needs of many bipolar patients" (Prien & Potter, 1990, p. 419). This view has been echoed by a number of other organizations including the American Psychiatric Association (2002), the British Association for Psychopharmacology, the World Federation of Societies of Biological Psychiatry (Jones et al., 2005a), the Royal Australian and New Zealand College of Psychiatrists (2004), and the United Kingdom's National Institute for Health and Clinical Excellence (2006).

Goodwin and Jamison (1990) illustrated this point on an individual level with a quote from a person with bipolar disorder, who stated:

> Lithium prevents my seductive but disastrous highs, diminishes my depressions, clears out the wool and webbing from my disordered thinking, slows me down . . . keeps me out of a hospital, alive and makes psychotherapy possible. But ineffably, psychotherapy *heals*. It makes some sense of the confusion, reins in the terrifying thoughts and feelings, returns some control and hope and opens the possibility of learning from it all. Pills cannot, do not *ease* one back into reality; they only bring one back headlong, careening, and faster than can be endured at times . . . No pills can help me deal with the problem of not wanting to take pills; likewise, no amount of analysis alone can prevent my manias and depressions. I need both (p. 725).

An impressive evidence base is emerging for psychological interventions for bipolar disorder, and while still at an early phase of development, recent research has indicated that CBT specifically, in combination with medication, can impact positively on symptoms, medication adherence, social functioning, and risk of relapse. Key elements of the underlying theoretical model will be described in Chapter 1.

As a result of the growing interest and research into psychological treatments, there are a number of excellent manuals and self-help books describing interventions for adults with bipolar disorder (Lam et al., 1999; Scott, 2001; Jones et al., 2002; Miklowitz, 2002; Newman et al., 2002; Bauer & McBride, 2003; Johnson & Leahy, 2004; Colom, 2006; Frank, 2007; Ramirez-Basco & Rush, 2007). However, none of these are designed specifically for use with a young population that is early in the course of the disorder. This is an important issue, given that onset of the disorder most commonly occurs during adolescence or early adulthood, and this is arguably the phase that offers the best opportunity for effective intervention.

This manual represents the work of the mania team at EPPIC in Melbourne, Australia, in conjunction with Professor Jan Scott, a leading researcher in the field of psychological therapies for bipolar disorder. It marks the development of a specialized psychosocial intervention for use with people in the early phase of the disorder.

EPPIC is a state-government-funded, public health unit, which treats people who are aged between 15 and 25 years and are experiencing a first-episode psychotic disorder. The mania team emerged within the unit to specialize in providing interventions for young people in the early phase of bipolar disorder with psychotic symptoms.

When we first began looking at providing psychosocial intervention for this population, we noted two main shortcomings in much of the existing literature, and it is primarily in response to these that we designed the intervention described in this manual. Firstly, there are no current manuals that address the unique challenges and opportunities presented by the young, first-episode population. Secondly, there often appears to be a marked discrepancy between the efficacy of interventions for bipolar disorder as reported in research trials, and the effectiveness of the same interventions in clinical settings with naturalistic clinical populations.

It is notable that many studies examining the effectiveness of psychological interventions in bipolar disorder tend to exclude people under the age of 18. Individuals with rapid cycling subtype, psychotic symptoms, current manic symptoms, comorbid Axis II diagnoses (including borderline or antisocial personality disorder), suicidal ideation or intent, illicit substance or excessive alcohol use, inability to read or write, or poor medication adherence are also typically excluded (Scott et al., 2001; Ball et al., 2003; Lam et al., 2005; Feeny et al., 2006; Scott et al., 2006). These criteria would exclude most of the population with whom we – and the majority of other clinical services throughout the world – work.

Such exclusion criteria are not limited to psychotherapy outcome literature, with Scott (2008) reporting that trials looking at the long-term efficacy of medications for relapse prevention are usually representative of no more than 10–15% of "real world" clients. Similarly, trials of acute treatments also use highly selected samples, with Zimmerman et al. (2005) reporting that 79% of a population of 599 depressed patients presenting at an outpatient clinic would be excluded from most antidepressant efficacy trials. Zimmerman and colleagues found specifically that while a number of these patients would be excluded due to their symptoms being rated as too mild, a significant subgroup would be excluded due to severity markers, including current suicidal ideation or intent, comorbid anxiety disorders, or substance use. The excluded participants with comorbidity were also found to be "a more chronically ill group, with more previous episodes, greater social and occupational impairment, and more personality pathology" (p. 1372).

Guscott and Taylor (1994) have named this difference between outcomes in a selected research population and typical cases seen in clinical practice, the "efficacy-effectiveness gap." In everyday practice, clinicians have to consider how they apply the findings of research studies to their clients and take this "gap" into account. Having had the opportunity to use cognitive behavioral approaches with a representative population of individuals with bipolar disorder across the age spectrum, we have selected the chapters for this book on the basis of the most commonly encountered problems in adolescents and young adults when they present or are diagnosed with bipolar disorder. As the field is continually developing, we realize that the core sections may be revised at a later date. However, we have chosen the issues that are most relevant to young people whilst trying to avoid replicating all the components covered in the standard CBT manuals for older adults (e.g. Newman et al., 2002).

A significant aim of this manual is to describe an intervention that was developed through our experience of working with a naturalistic, "real world" population of young people who were experiencing their first episode of mania and who had previously had little, if any, contact with mental health services. The majority of our young people presented with comorbid conditions and complex difficulties. Furthermore, "psychological mindedness," motivation, or even engagement with health services was neither presupposed nor common.

In conclusion, the aim of this manual is to describe a psychological intervention that is effective for working with young people with bipolar disorder, and which addresses the specific developmental issues relating to this population. While recognizing there is currently a sparse research literature on psychological interventions for young people with bipolar disorder, we have drawn from research on interventions for adults with bipolar disorder, the adolescent depression literature, literature describing key concepts in early intervention, and literature describing interventions for young people with psychotic disorders. As we are aware of the risks of extrapolating from other areas of research, we have been careful to include only interventions that we have found to be clinically effective.

Our intervention broadly utilizes a CBT orientation, but the complexity and hetero-geneity of this population requires a flexible model. Therefore our intervention also draws from solution-focused, narrative, client-centered, cognitive analytic, social rhythm, and family therapies.

Bipolar disorder

Moods are so essential to our navigating the world that when they go awry it is only a matter of time until distress and disaster hit. Moods allow us to gauge people and circumstance, alert us to danger and opportunity, and provide us with the means to convey our emotional and physical state to others.

Jamison (2003, p. xv)

Bipolar disorder, also known as manic depression, is a mood disorder that can involve extreme changes in affect, cognition, and behavior. In its extreme form, bipolar disorder can be associated with psychotic symptoms and can require inpatient admission due to disorganization and impulsivity in the manic phase, or due to suicidal ideation or neglect of self-care in the depressive phase. It affects males and females in equal numbers, and has similar rates across all socio-economic groups. Its onset generally occurs during late adolescence or early adulthood, with this having significant implications for the person's developmental trajectory and quality of life. This will be described later in the chapter.

While the *Diagnostic and Statistical Manual of Mental Disorders: Fourth Edition – Text Revision* (DSM-IV-TR) (American Psychiatric Association, 2000) should be consulted regarding diagnosis, a brief summary is as follows:

- A major depressive episode is diagnosed through the presence of depressed mood or loss of interest or pleasure for most of the day, nearly every day for two weeks or more. It must also be accompanied by five or more from nine symptoms, including feelings of worthlessness or guilt, insomnia or hypersomnia, psychomotor agitation or retardation, and fatigue.
- A manic episode is diagnosed through the presence of elevated, expansive, or irritable mood lasting at least one week, and of three or more from seven additional symptoms (or four or more if the mood is only irritable) including inflated self-esteem, increased talkativeness, reduced need for sleep, flight of ideas, and an increase in goal-directed activity.
- Hypomania can be seen as a milder form of mania. It draws from the same list of seven symptoms as mania, but symptoms only need to have been present for four days and cannot include psychotic symptoms. It does not require hospitalization or cause marked impairment in social or occupational functioning.
- A mixed episode occurs when a person meets criteria for both a manic episode and a major depressive episode nearly every day for at least one week, and when the disrupted mood causes a significant level of impairment in functioning.

The DSM-IV-TR defines four main subtypes of bipolar disorder:

- Bipolar I disorder, in which the person must have experienced at least one manic episode.
- Bipolar II disorder, where the person has had one or more depressive episodes, and at least one hypomanic episode, with no manic or mixed episodes.

- Cyclothymic disorder, where for at least two years, the person has had numerous periods of hypomania and depressive symptoms that do not meet criteria for a major depressive episode, and has not been without these for more than two months at a time.
- Bipolar disorder not otherwise specified, which can include very rapid alternation of manic and depressive symptoms, which meet symptom criteria but not minimum duration.

It is notable that clients do not always present with symptoms that fit classic textbook descriptions, and this is especially true in the early stages of bipolar disorder. Many researchers in the field describe the concept of bipolar *spectrum* disorders, which encapsulates the various manifestations of disorders that do not fit the criteria for bipolar I disorder, but nevertheless seem to be part of this diagnostic grouping. As young people often present with variations of the classic symptoms or syndromes (a cluster of symptoms that usually co-occur) of bipolar disorder, this topic will be described further in Chapter 2.

Clinical descriptions of manic and depressive symptoms have a long history. For example, in the first century AD, in his book *On the Causes and Symptoms of Chronic Diseases*, Arataeus gave a description of different types of manic symptoms which could still apply today. He noted: "Some patients with mania are cheerful – they laugh, play, dance day and night, and stroll through the market, sometimes with a garland on their head, as if they had won a game: these patients do not worry their relatives. But others fly into a rage . . . the manifestations of mania are countless. Some manics, who are intelligent and well educated, deal with astronomy, although they never studied it, with philosophy, but autodidactically, they consider poetry the gift of muses" (Marneros & Goodwin, 2005, p. 5).

While bipolar disorder is generally thought to affect around 1.6% of the population (Kessler et al., 1994; Bauer et al., 2002), there has been growing recognition of the concept of a spectrum between unipolar depression and bipolar disorder (Phelps et al., 2008). Using a broader definition, between 3.5% and 6% of people may experience some form of the disorder (Elgie & Morselli, 2007; Merikangas et al., 2007).

Given its prevalence, persistence, and the degree of impairment that can be associated with bipolar disorder, it should not come as a surprise to note that it is rated the sixth leading cause of disability among all types of physical or mental health disorders in people aged 19–40 (Murray & Lopez, 1996), a higher position than schizophrenia. In financial terms, Begley et al. (2001) calculated that the lifetime cost of all people developing bipolar disorder in the United States in 1998 was $24 billion, with average costs ranging from $11 720 for a person experiencing a single manic episode, to $624 785 for a person with multiple episodes. Furthermore, it has been estimated that an adult developing bipolar disorder in his/her mid-twenties effectively loses 9 years of life expectancy, 12 years of normal health, and 14 years of work activity (Prien & Potter, 1990).

Historically it has been suggested that whilst bipolar disorder has the potential to be recurrent with high rates of relapse, most individuals experience good inter-episode recovery. However, this was challenged by a prospective study of 146 people with bipolar I disorder, which found that participants were symptomatic for over 47% of the 13-year follow-up period (Judd et al., 2002). The percentage of time spent in each phase of the disorder is illustrated in Figure 1.1. Joffe et al. (2004) reported similar findings in their study, which found that bipolar participants experienced depressive symptoms for 40.9% and manic symptoms for 6% of the time during a follow-up period of almost 3 years.

In addition to poor inter-episode recovery, bipolar disorder has one of the highest lifetime risks for suicide associated with any psychiatric disorder, with research indicating that between 15% and 20% of people with the disorder take their own lives (Goodwin & Jamison, 1990). Notably, the suicide rate in bipolar disorder has been found to be almost

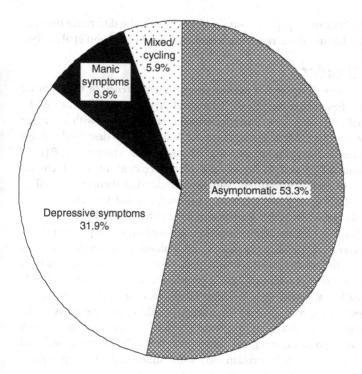

Figure 1.1 Breakdown of time spent in various phases of bipolar disorder. Data taken from Judd et al., 2002.

double that of unipolar depression (Chen & Dilsaver, 1996; Mitchell & Malhi, 2004). Encouragingly, however, a long-term naturalistic follow-up demonstrated that receiving treatment is associated with lower suicide rates and lower mortality rates from all causes compared with not receiving treatment (Angst et al., 2002).

Difficulties associated with bipolar disorder

A number of difficulties have been found to be associated with bipolar disorder, including:

- Adjustment problems have been noted to affect a number of people in the initial phase of bipolar disorder. For example, Goodwin and Jamison (1990) found that on discovering the disorder may be chronic and recurrent, many people reported experiencing ambivalence, anxiety, disappointment, denial, and anger.
- Financial difficulties have been reported by 70% of people with bipolar disorder and their partners, with these often remaining long-term (Targum et al., 1981).
- Poor self-esteem is highly prevalent, with evidence that people with bipolar disorder may view themselves as different or defective, even when asymptomatic (Rush, 1988).
- Even when in remission, people with bipolar disorder have been found to have poorer social adjustment when compared with control participants (Blairy et al., 2004).
- Coryell et al. (1993) summarized: "The psychosocial impairment associated with mania and major depression extends to essentially all areas of functioning and persists for years, even among individuals who experience sustained resolution of clinical symptoms" (p. 720). While Coryell and colleagues may be describing the more severe end of the bipolar spectrum, it is nevertheless notable that the disorder can have a negative impact on a significant number of people with the diagnosis.

However, even with mounting evidence of the potential difficulties associated with bipolar disorder, many people remain untreated, with a recent World Health Organization bulletin estimating that the "treatment gap" for bipolar disorder (i.e. the difference between those experiencing the disorder and those receiving treatment) was 56% (Kohn et al., 2004).

Etiology of bipolar disorder

The search for causes of bipolar disorder has existed since the emergence of the disorder itself. The ancient Greeks believed that mood and behavioral disturbances were caused by imbalances in our essential body fluids or "humors" (Evans et al., 2003), with a similar concept being promoted by the physician Alcmaeon (around 500 BC), who described sadness as being related to the interaction between bile and the brain (Angst & Marneros, 2001).

Until recently, the dominant models of bipolar disorder have continued to focus on biological factors, specifically neurotransmitters and neuroendocrine theories as well as considerable debate about the role of genetic factors. However, the last few decades have also seen a greater emphasis placed on stress-diathesis models of bipolar disorder (Prien & Potter, 1990; Scott, 1995; Scott & Colom, 2005). Like the literature on schizophrenia, there has been an increasing acknowledgement that genetics and biological factors alone cannot account for the emergence of bipolar disorder and that psychosocial factors, such as personality or cognitive style, the experience of significant life events, and aspects of family environment such as negative affective style or high levels of expressed emotion, can increase the risk of relapse in bipolar disorder or adversely affect the prognosis of an episode. The current consensus is that a multi-factorial model offers the most robust explanation of the causes of bipolar disorder, no single gene is the "primary cause," and no psychological or social factor can fully explain why some individuals develop bipolar disorder whilst others, with the same genetic predisposition, do not.

As individuals who develop bipolar disorder and their families often ask about the possible causes, we now offer brief comments on some key issues in current biological research. We then highlight areas of interest in psychosocial research that are relevant to the clinical sections later in the book. This is not meant to be an exhaustive review of every current model, and we recognize that new findings will be published that will overtake some of the ideas discussed here, and that the psychobiosocial model will continue to evolve over the coming decades. Most importantly, the key "take-home" message is that individuals appear to inherit a "risk" of developing bipolar disorder and whether that risk is expressed or not (i.e. whether they manifest the symptoms of the disorder) will be determined by a number of psychobiosocial factors.

Genetic and biological models

Current research on etiology tends to maintain a strong biological focus, and a range of biological factors have been implicated in the causation of bipolar disorder. The strong familial clustering of cases gives an indication that inheritance (and therefore genes) plays a role in the causes of bipolar disorder, and research has identified several candidate genes which may be associated with the disorder, as well as specific loci that may confer risk (Abou Jamra et al., 2007; Kato, 2007; Sklar et al., 2008).

Twin studies have generally shown that if one twin has bipolar disorder, the risk in the co-twin is much higher than expected by chance. For example, Berrettini (2000) reported that concordance rates were 14% for dizygotic twins (who have half their genes in common) and 65% for monozygotic twins (who are genetically identical). However, whilst the levels of concordance clearly indicate that genetic factors are important, the fact that in many pairs only one identical twin manifests the disorder indicates that genes alone cannot explain the variance. As Bauer and McBride (2003) succinctly concluded, "Thus, it is impossible ...

that manic depressive disorder is totally genetically determined" (p. 38). Furthermore, results of studies investigating genetics in bipolar disorder are generally not consistent with the notion of a single causative gene for the disorder. Therefore, it appears likely that the contribution of genetics to etiology is through a complex interaction of a number of genes and the environment (Hyman, 1999).

As in other mood disorders, neurotransmitter abnormalities and dysfunctional neuro-endocrine stress responses have also been implicated in the onset and/or outcome of bipolar disorder. The main weakness of such models is the absence of a robust theory that explains why changes lead to mania in some circumstances and depression in others. Research focusing on neurotransmitters has shown a deficiency in norepinephrine in people with depressed mood, and changes in serotonin and dopamine have been linked with manic and psychotic symptoms (Zubieta et al., 2000).

Recent promising work on neural pathways has identified reduced activation of the dorsolateral prefrontal cortex and orbitofrontal cortex, and increased activity in the amygdala in adults with bipolar disorder (for a review see Pavuluri, 2004). Similarly, a review by Malhi et al. (2004) cited research indicating reduced prefrontal and subgenual cingulate volumes, and enlargement of subcortical and medial temporal structures such as the basal ganglia and amygdala, in people with bipolar disorder. These circuits are import-ant, as changes in their functioning may explain some of the changes in mood and activation observed in bipolar disorder and perhaps tentatively help us understand why atypical antipsychotic medications (which act predominantly on dopamine pathways) appear to be useful in treating acute bipolar episodes and stabilizing an individual's mental state. Furthermore, they form part of the behavioral activation system, which, through its role in rewards and goal-directed behavior, is now seen as an important potential pathway linking life events, cognitive style, and brain activity with onset of mood episodes.

Neurobiological research in bipolar disorder has also found increases in the volume of the lateral brain ventricles (Swayze et al., 1990), while other studies have noted increased binding cells in the thalamus and ventral brain stem (Zubieta et al., 2000). Inconsistent results have been observed in temporal lobe studies, and there has been some indication that hippocampal volume may also contribute to the etiology of bipolar disorder (Frey et al., 2007). A difficulty with much of this research is whether these changes are a cause or a consequence of the mental disorder.

Psychosocial models of bipolar disorder

Despite the strong historical research focus on exploring biological and genetic etiological pathways to bipolar disorder, there is emerging evidence that life events, stress (including family stress and high expressed emotion), and cognitive style can influence the course of bipolar disorder, especially the likelihood of relapse. The exact role of these factors in the onset of the first episode is less clear cut, but there is increasing evidence that psychosocial stressors can precipitate the onset of symptoms so that an underlying vulnerability to bipolar disorder becomes manifest in those at risk (Scott, 2003).

There is currently a complex literature describing potential psychosocial mechanisms relating to bipolar disorder, and a detailed analysis of each theory is beyond the scope of this manual. We will therefore focus on a brief description of the evolution of the concept of the "manic defense" and its recent reformulations and then highlight some more recent cognitive models that together inform the integrative model we use in our clinical work. Interested readers should also refer to Healy and Williams (1989) or Scott (2003) for a review of cognitive models, and Power's (2005) excellent overview of currently dominant psychosocial models. These models generally share the view that specific cognitive styles, when interacting with life events and biological vulnerability, may increase the likelihood of developing manic or depressive symptoms, and that exacerbation of these symptoms is in turn further driven by underlying beliefs and attributions about the meaning of the early symptoms experienced by an individual.

The "manic defense," self-esteem and bipolar disorder

Research describing the contribution of psychological factors to the onset and course of bipolar disorder has a long history. In 1911, Karl Abraham suggested that rather than being polar opposites, mania and depression "are dominated by the same complexes, and that it is only the patient's attitudes to these complexes that is different" (Bentall, 2003, p. 277). At this time, the concept of the "manic defense" emerged. Klein (1974) provided a succinct definition that "mania is a massive defence arising from the failure of the containing processes which normally occur in the infant-mother relationship, and which results in a catastrophic fragmentation of the ego" (p. 261). Bateman et al. (1954) provided another psychoanalytic conceptualization of mania, which focused on the role of trauma. They suggested that past or present trauma can result in guilt, which is avoided or defended against by "desperate vigilance and by a psychologic counteroffensive which is no longer consistent with reality" (p. 353). They further commented: "It is not sufficient for the manic merely to avoid painful recollections or stimuli. He must actively evade, repudiate, or counter-attack them. Therefore, the manic mood is one of extreme tenseness" (p. 353). They concluded: "All the symptoms, in addition to serving the essential manic aim, also serve a secondary aim of protecting the patient from external interference while he is engaged in his attempt at regaining psychic equilibrium" (p. 356).

In the 1960s, the rise of the biological model of bipolar disorder and the emphasis on treatment with medications overshadowed psychological theories, and the potential implications of the manic defense received less attention. This was compounded by the revolution in psychology with cognitive and behavioral models that were amenable to empirical testing being favored over psychoanalytic theories, which at times also defied easy comprehension (e.g. Morgenson, 1996). Studies that explored self-esteem and, later, social desirability and self-representations, also began to appear. For example, Winters and Neale (1985) wrote a highly influential article in which they hypothesized that although research participants with remitted bipolar disorder did not usually *report* impaired self-esteem, they may nevertheless have *experienced* cognitive schema relating to low self-esteem. Winters and Neale used the Pragmatic Inference Test (PIT), an implicit measure of self-esteem in which participants are given ambiguous stories (such as a person becoming unemployed or a first date going badly) and are then asked to attribute why the event occurred. They found that, even when in remission, people with a history of bipolar disorder or unipolar depression were significantly more likely than control participants to attribute unsuccessful outcomes to factors relating to the person. One implication of this finding is that people prone to bipolar disorder or unipolar depression may be more likely to blame themselves following a negative event rather than look to external environmental factors. Winters and Neale concluded that participants with bipolar disorder might have negative feelings about the self that were not revealed on the typical, explicit self-report measures employed in research settings.

The findings of Winters and Neale (2005) have been replicated by Lyon et al. (1999), who also observed that while manic participants were more likely to *endorse* positive words as being descriptive of themselves (e.g. "successful," "capable," and "valuable"), similarly to bipolar depressive participants, they were more likely to *recall* negative words (e.g. "deficient," "unloved," and "weak"). The authors suggested that these findings – which utilized implicit rather than explicit measures – also appear to support the concept of mania serving a defensive function against poor self-esteem, and occurring beyond the person's awareness.

Neale (1988) proposed that *unstable* self-esteem coupled with unreasonable standards for success may be predisposing factors for bipolar disorder. Although there is little empirical support for this hypothesis, Pardoen and colleagues' (1993) study of self-esteem confirmed the presence of social conformism in people with bipolar disorder. Furthermore, recent research has shown that people with bipolar disorder often indicate lower self-esteem on more subtle or implicit measures, possibly as some core beliefs or schemas occur outside the person's conscious awareness (Timbremont & Braet, 2004). A key methodological lesson from these studies is the need to consider the use of implicit as well as explicit measures of cognitive style (Bentall, 2003).

Recent studies on levels of self-esteem in bipolar disorder suggest variations may also be a function of lability as well as differences between implicit and explicit ratings (Scott, 2003). Scott and colleagues have identified that labile self-esteem, rather than a fixed low level of self-esteem, may potentially differentiate people with bipolar disorder from people with severe unipolar disorders in the depressed or euthymic phases of disorder. However, unstable self-esteem and low levels of self-esteem are both known to confer similar levels of risk for depressive relapse (Kernis et al., 1993).

This research has led to a number of theorists, including Bentall (2003), revisiting the concept of the manic defense and adapting it to a more contemporary cognitive model, whereby the person may be protected from a poor or fluctuating self-esteem and a strong need for approval from others by grandiose beliefs and elevated mood.

Thomas et al. (2007) also supported the hypothesis that mania can result from a coping style which attempts to avoid negative emotion. They found that manic participants – compared with depressed bipolar participants, remitted bipolar participants, and non-bipolar controls – showed higher levels of risk-taking and active coping. They summarized: "Although the findings provide support for a version of the depression-avoidance hypothesis, the mechanism proposed here is simpler than that proposed by psychoanalytic theorists" (p. 251). They concluded that excessive distraction may overload the behavioral activation system, and that disruption of circadian rhythms may contribute to the etiology of mania.

Stressful life events, "daily hassles" and circadian rhythm disruption in bipolar disorder

Several studies have implicated stress and life events in the initial onset and relapse of bipolar disorder. For example, Bebbington et al. (1993) found that, compared with control participants, people developing bipolar disorder experienced significantly more critical life events, particularly in the three months prior to their first episode. This pattern remained even when incidents that may have been related to the disorder itself were removed. Similar findings have been reported by Kennedy et al. (1983), Frank et al. (2000), and Hammen and Gitlin (1997). A prospective study by Ellicott et al. (1990) found that individuals with bipolar disorder who had experienced a high number of stressful life events were in excess of four times more likely to relapse than those who had not encountered similar stressors. A meta-analysis by Altman et al. (2006) concluded: "The majority of research in the field, in both small and large studies, supports the notion that stressful life events have an overall negative impact on outcomes in bipolar disorder, both in terms of contributing to relapse and in lengthening time to recovery" (p. 273). Furthermore, research in both circadian rhythms (Hlastala et al., 2000) and neurobiology (Post, 1992) has indicated that people who have had fewer episodes, and young people specifically, may be even more vulnerable to bipolar disorder in response to life events.

A large study involving 1565 individuals with bipolar disorder and 16 200 age- and gender-matched controls (Kessing et al., 2004) was able to elucidate the relative importance of some specific life events in bipolar disorder. This study found that the suicide of a mother or sibling significantly increased the risk of a first admission for a manic or mixed episode by 5.75 and 4.7 times respectively. Recent unemployment and divorce both increased the likelihood of a first admission by 1.5 times, and marriage in the previous year almost doubled the risk of first admission.

However, rather than focusing solely on the importance of significant life events, some recent research on young people has examined "daily hassles" – including everyday annoyances such as minor arguments or disagreements – and their influence on mood and behavior. Dumont and Provost (1999) suggested that focusing on daily hassles may allow for more subjective analysis, which more closely reflects people's experiences than objective measures. Secondly, they noted that "life events are relatively rare, whereas daily hassles are common and show a greater interindividual variance" (p. 345). Finally, they suggested that research has shown that daily hassles have a greater influence on mental health difficulties than life events. They concluded: "This implies that daily hassles might be better predictors of the psychological health of young adolescents than are life events" (p. 345). This is supported in research by Thompson et al. (2007), who measured plasma cortisol levels in young people at high risk of developing psychotic disorders, as this has been found to correlate with symptoms of anxiety and depression. They reported that while there was no correlation between cortisol levels and significant stressful life events, there was a positive correlation between cortisol levels and the number of day-to-day hassles reported by the young person.

There has been some debate as to the mechanism by which stressful life events or daily hassles could lead to onset and relapse in bipolar disorder. One suggestion is that this occurs through the impact of such events on circadian rhythms, with disruption to these having long been suspected as playing a part in the development of bipolar disorder and relapse. For example, Malkoff-Schwartz et al. (1998) reported that stressful life events that involved social disruption were associated with the onset of manic episodes, regardless of the episode's severity. Interestingly, however, *severely* stressful life events, regardless of their level of social disruption, have been correlated with the onset of manic and depressive episodes (Frank et al., 2000). As Satterfield (1999) succinctly described in a paper on rapid-cycling bipolar disorder, "life events disrupt critical social rhythms and push biologically and affectively vulnerable ... patients into a cascading state of biological and affective dysregulation" (p. 359).

A specific aspect of circadian rhythms that has attracted significant attention has been the area of sleep. Colombo et al. (1999) found that 10% of people with bipolar disorder developed manic or hypomanic symptoms after induced sleep deprivation. A recent prospective study by Meyer and Maier (2006) specifically examined the role of sleep patterns in young people. They found that those at risk of bipolar disorder did not differ in their *amount* of sleep, compared to control participants and people at risk of unipolar depression, but did differ on their *regularity* of sleep and daily activities. Meyer and Maier concluded: "From a theoretical as well as empirical point of view, there is reason to assume that circadian rhythms play a central role in the origin and course of bipolar disorders" (p. 104). Even subtle changes in sleep and biological rhythms may be clinically meaningful, with Berk et al. (2008a) having found a significant increase in suicide rates in a national sample after transition to daylight saving, which alters sleep rhythms by only one hour.

Johnson (2005) reported that life events significantly affected speed of relapse and length of time for recovery from both manic and depressive episodes. However, Johnson differentiated between the type of events experienced by the person and the polarity of their mood. Specifically, manic episodes were more likely to be affected by events that upset circadian rhythms and involved goal attainment, while depressive episodes tended to be related to negative life events.

While circadian rhythm disruption offers one possible etiological factor, the mechanism by which life events affect mood has been subject to considerable discussion. Scott (2003) noted that cognitive changes and sometimes mood elevation may occur following sleep disruption, but whether isolated manic symptoms then cascade into a full-blown episode depends on whether the individual makes dispositional or situational attributions. Healy and Williams (1989) provided the example, "this efficiency and speed is due to my natural intuition and intelligence," leading to actions that increase rather than decrease the risk of manic relapse. Other researchers conceptualize bipolar disorder as occurring due to individuals having "impaired shock absorbers," in which the person's ability to "cushion" the impact of positive or negative events is less effective than that of people who do not have bipolar disorder. A literature review by Johnson (2005) concluded: "Even when they are euthymic, people with bipolar disorder appear to experience frequent and intense emotions in response to environmental conditions" (p. 251).

Bentall (2003) reported a model similar to the "impaired shock absorber" theory, describing an "excitability hypothesis" in which people with bipolar disorder experience a dysregulation of behavioral activation, and crave social contact, excitement, and motor activity. He found that people with bipolar disorder endorsed questionnaire items including "when good things happen to me, it affects me strongly" and "I will often do things for no other reason than that they might be fun" (p. 289). Bentall (2003) elaborated by suggesting that when people with bipolar disorder experience negative life events, this interacts with a basic underlying dysphoria and a pessimistic attributional style, which may lead to depression. However, if combined with distraction or high levels of behavioral activation – such as becoming involved in risk-taking behavior and drive to succeed – the resulting excitement and circadian rhythm disruption (i.e. changes in eating patterns and sleep loss) can lead to mania.

It is also important to note the importance of the bidirectional nature of stress, coping, and mood, as stressors can impact on coping style, which may in turn result in the experience of more stress and altered mood. Most notably, coping strategies such as substance use or social withdrawal – while potentially an attempt to reduce short-term stress – appear likely to result in further difficulties and exacerbation of mood symptoms.

Cognitive style and bipolar disorder

While the relationship between life events and mood is complex, a mediating factor appears to be attributional style, and a number of researchers (e.g. Lam et al., 1999; Bentall, 2003; Johnson & Leahy, 2004; Ramirez-Basco & Rush, 2007) have described models for understanding bipolar disorder within a cognitive behavioral framework. Pioneering work was conducted by Aaron Beck (1976), who noted that many people with depression appeared to have characteristic ways of thinking which were either inaccurate or unhelpful. Specifically,

Beck defined the "negative cognitive triad," in which a person with depression will select-ively attend to, and recall more easily, information which fits with their negative views of themselves, the world, and the future. According to Beck's model, this way of thinking impacts on the person's emotional state and behavior, which in turn impacts further on the person's negative thinking. Beck further described the bidirectional interaction between this thinking style and the environment, as people may actually find themselves failing at tasks or relationships, being criticized or withdrawing socially as a result of their impaired performance, which in turn could lead to further negative cognitions in a downward spiral of mood, behavior, and cognition. More recently, Lyon et al. (1999) similarly concluded: "Bipolar depression, like unipolar depression, appears to be characterised by a negative self-schema, a corresponding tendency to blame the self for negative experiences, and selective attention to depression-related stimuli" (p. 279).

Beck et al. (2006) noted that, similar to the negative cognitive triad common in people with depression, people prone to mania tend to hold clusters of *positive* beliefs about the self ("I am strong"), relationships ("everybody loves me"), pleasure/excitement ("I have to live for today"), and activity ("I have enough energy to do anything I want to") (p. 239). In Beck's model, mania may be a mirror image of depression, being associated with cognitive distor-tions such as jumping to positive conclusions, underestimating risks, minimizing problems, and overvaluing immediate gratification. In addition, positive experiences may be selectively attended to and recalled more easily, with negative events being minimized or ignored.

However, as elated mania is only one form of mania, it is also clear that further elaboration of cognitive models is required to explain dysphoric mania and mixed states (Scott, 2003). Furthermore, some researchers have suggested that rather than manic and depressive cognitions being polar opposites, they in fact share some similarities at the level of core beliefs or schemas, particularly in relation to the experience of poor self-esteem (Scott et al., 2000; Schwannauer, 2003). Ginsberg (1979) also suggested that the two disorders are similar, stating: "Mania does not end depression, it interrupts it" (p. 8).

Johnson (2005) observed that, compared with control participants, people with bipolar I disorder and students who were vulnerable to hypomania tended to have higher expect-ations of success, and were more likely to choose more difficult goals when given a choice of tasks. Furthermore, Johnson found that when experiencing a manic episode, people were more able to recall positive events, and were more likely to pursue difficult tasks and ignore danger cues after experiencing small successes. Johnson noted: "High goal setting appears to be a stable characteristic among persons with bipolar disorder" (p. 254). One clinical implication of this is that if people with bipolar disorder hold high expectations, and are more likely to be encouraged by small successes, they may become more driven to complete tasks that would be abandoned by people without the disorder. On occasions when success does eventuate, this could contribute to an upward spiral of energy, confidence, and disruption to sleep, which could precipitate a manic episode.

A further cognitive factor which has been implicated in the development and mainten-ance of manic or depressive episodes is that of memory bias. A review by Johnson (2005) stated that mood state could provoke recall for specific memories, such as low mood being related to a preoccupation with memories of negative past experiences. Similar findings emerged in studies by Eich et al. (1994) and Weingartner et al. (1977), who found that when depressed, people could recall equal numbers of positive and negative memories, whereas when hypomanic, they would recall more than three times as many positive as negative experiences. Clearly, such biases can be seen to have a role in maintaining manic or depressive symptoms.

Schema and bipolar disorder

As noted above, there is considerable research relating attributional style to mood disorders. Scott et al. (2000) found that even when in remission, people with bipolar disorder scored significantly higher than control participants on the Dysfunctional Attitude Scale (DAS) (Weissman & Beck, 1978), a measure of negative core underlying beliefs. In other research utilizing the DAS, Power (2005) found that two specific subscales, namely "goal attainment" and "antidependency," appeared particularly relevant to bipolar disorder. Power suggested these attitudes may foster a "positive feedback loop" (p. 1107), where a person with a vulnerability to bipolar disorder will seek to enhance positive mood through goal-focused behavior while rejecting any negative feedback from others, with the consequence of increased goal-directed behavior leading to social rhythm disruption and increased likelihood of disordered mood.

Ball et al. (2003) also noted the importance of attribution and bipolar disorder, stating: "Cognitive and schematic vulnerabilities are seen to act as filters in triggering mood shifts when stressful life events occur" (p. 43). They elaborated: "Dependency and self criticism, interpersonal sensitivity, need for approval, and perfectionism have been found to be more prevalent in individuals with bipolar disorder than unipolar depression" (p. 43). Ball and colleagues concluded that a circular system can be established where personality factors could heighten an individual's vulnerability to bipolar disorder, but that unstable mood can then itself promote personality factors, such as dependency, which could then pre-dispose towards further episodes of mood difficulties. In addition, they also suggested that becoming symptomatic and experiencing bipolar disorder itself may "activate or heighten self-defeating constructs in vulnerable individuals" (p. 44).

We believe that understanding cognitive factors, including the role of schemas in the development of bipolar disorder, has significant implications for clinical work. While the literature on life events and circadian rhythms may help us understand one mechanism for the impact of specific incidents on mood, it does not allow for any more specificity as to which types of events are likely to precipitate bipolar episodes in which individuals. Better understanding of schemas as a mediator between an event and affective change may help us predict which types of events may make a person vulnerable to relapse.

For example, a review by Johnson et al. (2000) found that negative life events, low social support, and low self-esteem were predictive of bipolar depression, but that "goal-attainment life events" (such as passing an exam or gaining a new job), rather than simply positive events in general, were associated with elevated mood.

An important paper by Francis-Raniere et al. (2006) also offers an explanation of the mediating role schemas may play, and why specific life events may lead to mood disorder in some people on some occasions but not others. The "event-congruency hypothesis" proposed that when life events occur which are congruent with a person's personality style or schemas (specifically where this involves high self-criticism and high performance expectation), the person may be more vulnerable to either depression or mania. Francis-Raniere and colleagues found that non-congruent events were not predictive of manic or depressive episodes, and that this effect was more significant for people with bipolar disorder than for people with unipolar depression. So, for example, if a person has strong schemas related to abandonment or vulnerability, the death of a relative or breakup of a relationship may be particularly challenging and likely to lead to a significant mood episode. Another person who does not hold these schemas may not be as affected by these events but, due to unrelenting standards or perfectionistic schemas, may be vulnerable to a manic or depressive episode in response to significant exam or work stress. The clinical application of the event-congruency hypothesis is discussed in more detail in Chapter 5.

One criticism of the cognitive model is that negative thinking styles could simply be state markers of depression, and that it is in fact depression which causes maladaptive thinking styles. However, this theory has been challenged by a recent large prospective study that included over 12 000 women (Evans et al., 2005). In their study, Evans and colleagues found that the endorsement of negative self-schema statements, such as "if others knew the real me they would not like me" and "I avoid saying what I think for fear of being rejected" (p. 303), was predictive of depression up to three years later in women who were not depressed during the initial assessment. They concluded: "Negative self-schemas are stable patterns of thinking that confer long-term vulnerability to developing depression" (p. 305). However, there does not appear to be as convincing evidence regarding cognitive trait markers for mania (Mansell et al., 2005; Jones et al., 2005b).

Another recent study by Timbremont and Braet (2004) reported a similar finding amongst adolescents, and found that even when in remission, adolescents with histories of depression showed similar cognitive vulnerabilities to adolescents with current depression. Specifically, they found that both groups (i.e. currently depressed and in remission), "lacked positive information processing that is characteristic in never depressed children" (p. 432), and that "both groups were characterized by significantly less positive self-schemas compared to never depressed children" (p. 435). These findings may indicate trait vulnerability or represent a "post-episode scar," but in either scenario, making early attempts to improve adaptive processing and self-concept would undoubtedly be a beneficial strategy.

Summary of etiological factors

It appears that the traditional "nature versus nurture" debate has largely been superseded by a consensus view that there is a complex interaction of multiple psychobiosocial factors including environmental, developmental, biological, cognitive, and genetic factors in the etiology of bipolar disorder. Importantly, the literature supports the contribution of psychosocial factors in the etiology of bipolar disorder and it appears that psychosocial factors may have a strong impact on the course of the disorder.

In a comprehensive review, Alloy et al. (2005) – the team responsible for the highly influential Temple-Wisconsin prospective studies of cognitive vulnerability – stated: "The evidence relating current environmental factors (stressful life events, social support, expressed emotion) to the course of bipolar disorders has been fairly consistent. Although relatively few in number, the methodologically sound prospective studies suggest that similar to the case for unipolar depression, the occurrence of stressful events may contribute proximal risk to onsets and recurrences of mood episodes in individuals with bipolar disorders" (p. 1055). Furthermore, regarding the role of cognitive styles, Alloy and colleagues concluded: "There is considerable evidence that cognitive styles alone, and particularly in combination with relevant life events, prospectively predict the course of bipolar depression and more mixed evidence that they predict the course of bipolar mania/hypomania" (p. 1063).

Our model integrates a number of psychological theories and asserts that, in addition to biological and environmental factors, cognitive factors, including schemas, can play a significant role in the etiology and course of bipolar disorder in young people. This highlights that interventions that stabilize circadian and social rhythms and attempt to reduce the impact of – or avert – certain types of events, and methods of reducing rigid (often perfectionistic) responses to daily hassles, are extremely important in the management of bipolar disorder. The research described earlier in this chapter has identified that some cognitive styles, such as high goal setting and perfectionism, are common in the bipolar population generally, and may represent a risk factor for developing episodes of the disorder. Modifying such beliefs may help maximize the benefit of various treatment components, for example overcoming cognitive barriers to medication adherence. However, we also believe that specific idiosyncratic schemas can mediate life events and may have a predictive quality allowing clinicians to anticipate which situations may put the young person at more risk of relapse. Furthermore, associated behavioral changes, such as increased or decreased activity levels, avoidance, further stimulation-seeking, and circadian rhythm disruption can create a loop which may maintain or exacerbate the initial schemas and lead to the emergence of further mood episodes. Finally, attributions regarding the disorder itself, which are likely to relate to underlying schemas, such as "getting bipolar disorder just shows what a loser I am/how weak I am" or "I should be able to manage this without medication," can also influence its course and the young person's willingness to engage in treatment.

Clearly, therefore, providing psychological interventions that target and modify these beliefs and associated behaviors can diminish the impact of the disorder and reduce the likelihood of relapse.

Outcome studies of psychological interventions with bipolar disorder

Interventions for bipolar disorder have traditionally been somewhat overlooked in the psycho-social intervention literature (Jones & Tarrier, 2005), with Bentall (2003) suggesting that less psychological research has been conducted into mania than any other major psychiatric disorder. As a result of psychosocial intervention research in bipolar disorder being in its infancy, and the subsequent lack of a strong current evidence base, we recognize that some caution is required. Similarly, we recognize that the literature on psychological interventions is evolving, with some of the literature strongly advocating these approaches, while some is more cautious. However, in recent years some promising research has emerged on the use of psychological therapies, and particularly, individual and family-based CBT. We would direct readers to Cochran (1984), Perry et al. (1999), and Zaretsky et al. (1999) for further details.

More recently, randomized controlled trials have indicated that individual CBT can reduce the number of relapses and need for hospitalization, increase the time of inter-episode wellbeing, enhance global functioning (Scott et al., 2001; Lam et al., 2005), reduce the length of manic episodes, and improve social functioning, impulsivity, and problem-solving (Perry et al., 1999) in people with bipolar disorder.

Recent reviews have concluded that CBT can impact on symptoms, medication adherence, social functioning, and risk of relapse in bipolar disorder (Huxley et al., 2000; Gonzalez-Pinto et al., 2004; Jones 2004; Scott & Gutierrez, 2004). A review by Alloy et al. (2005) concluded that, despite some methodological limitations, available evidence indicates that psychosocial treatments attending to social rhythms, reducing stress, family communication skills, and cognitive principles "show great promise as adjuncts to pharmacotherapy for bipolar disorder" (p. 1068).

A recent, multi-centre, randomized controlled trial by Miklowitz et al. (2007a) compared CBT, family-focused therapy (FFT), and interpersonal and social rhythm therapy (IPSRT). All three treatments were found to be superior to collaborative care, which consisted of three 50-minute sessions involving a psychoeducational videotape and workbook. Interestingly, there were no differences in outcome between the three active therapies. Miklowitz and colleagues acknowledged that the study may have been underpowered to detect differences between groups, but also concluded: "The lack of statistically significant differences between the intensive modalities (i.e. CBT, IPSRT, and FFT) may also reflect the effect of shared components of the treatments, which are in many ways more striking than their differences" (p. 425).

The largest randomized controlled trial of cognitive therapy for bipolar disorder to date, which included 253 participants, showed that CBT appeared to offer no benefit over treatment as usual in terms of recurrence of symptoms (Scott et al., 2006). However, *post hoc* analysis yielded an important finding, namely that the number of episodes the person had experienced significantly impacted on the effectiveness of therapy. Specifically, the fewer episodes the person had experienced, the higher the likelihood that the therapy would be successful. This clearly has implications for the importance of early intervention, and would indicate that the most efficacious time to provide psychological therapy is early in the course of the disorder. Colom (2008) conducted a *post hoc* analysis of his trial of psychoeducation in bipolar disorder, and also found some support for the notion of greater response earlier in the course of the disorder.

Three recent papers have described psychological interventions for young people with bipolar disorder. The first of these studies was that of Pavuluri et al. (2004), who reported preliminary evidence for their 'child and family-focused CBT' for pediatric bipolar disorder. Danielson et al. (2004) described a CBT intervention for adolescents with bipolar disorder that comprised a 12-session acute intervention with booster sessions. Effectiveness outcomes from this intervention were later reported in pilot study data by Feeny et al. (2006). With the exception of these papers, research advocating psychological interventions for young people with bipolar disorder remains largely neglected.

However, there have been a number of studies examining psychological interventions for young people with unipolar depression, with a review by Curry (2001) stating: "Previous reviews have indicated that cognitive behavior therapy (CBT) has been the most frequently investigated treatment for depression in young people and that it has received the most empirical support" (p. 1091). This would indicate that CBT can be effective in work with young people with mood disorders, but clearly emphasizes the need for further research on psychological interventions involving a young bipolar population.

Developmental aspects of bipolar disorder in young people

That the illness should develop in adult life without recognizable precursors in childhood seems as improbable as Athena's springing fully formed from the brow of Zeus.

Kestenbaum (1982, p. 246)

While there are not necessarily always childhood precursors, a recent large survey by Hirschfeld et al. (2003) found that 59% of respondents with bipolar disorder reported that their first symptoms occurred in childhood and adolescence. Most recent studies have found that bipolar disorder generally has its onset in adolescence, specifically between the ages of 15 and 19 (Burke et al., 1990; Lish et al., 1994; Hilty et al., 1999), and Begley et al. (2001) reported that around 98% of people who develop bipolar disorder do so before the age of 25.

The fact that onset generally occurs during adolescence has a number of important implications, as adolescence is widely recognized as a crucial developmental stage involving significant cognitive, emotional, social, and physical (including hormonal and neurological) changes (Steinberg, 1987; Seiffgre-Krenke, 2000; Corsano et al., 2006). Specifically, it has been noted that adolescence is a time associated with consolidation of identity, development of sexual and close peer relationships, setting and achieving educational and vocational goals, development of empathy and awareness of others' needs, delaying immediate gratification, increasing autonomy, separating from parents, and taking increased responsibility for behavior (Hill, 1983; Jackson et al., 1999).

There has been recognition in the literature for some time that adolescence can be a time associated with significant upheaval for some people. For example, in their longitudinal study of 59 non-clinical adolescents, Golombek et al. (1989) concluded that "turmoil is not universal to adolescent development" but "two-thirds of teenagers do demonstrate some upheaval in personality functions at some point during their development" (p. 503).

Developing any significant disorder during late teens and early adulthood can be particularly challenging due to its potential impact on achieving developmental milestones, particularly that of attaining independence. At this developmental stage, many young people may be moving out of home, gaining financial independence, completing school, finding employment or undertaking tertiary study, and developing intimate relationships. However, for young people in the early phase of bipolar disorder, disorganization, hospitalization, and the impact of the disorder on social, emotional, and cognitive functioning may delay all of these goals, and create further distress when the young person compares their perceived achievements to those of their peers.

Waters and Calleia (1983) stated that the development of bipolar disorder in adolescence could result in the "absence of a stable internal milieu" (p. 184). Clearly, disruption to basic vital functions including energy, sleep, confidence, appetite, and ability to concentrate, can result in a person having difficulty forming an idea of who they are, at a crucial time in their identity formation. In describing first-episode psychosis, Jackson et al. (1999) reported: "The effects . . . on the self and development may be potentially cataclysmic, causing derailment, truncation, deflection or paralysis of the person's developmental trajectory" (p. 271). This appears equally applicable for people experiencing first-episode bipolar disorder.

It is also important to note the impact of bipolar disorder on individuation and role within the family. Onset of bipolar disorder at this important developmental stage may result in family members needing to take an increased, rather than reduced, role in the young person's life, which can be particularly challenging. Both poles of bipolar disorder may result in carers having to monitor the young person more closely and having to take more directive roles. For example, in the manic phase, carers may need to attempt to control and limit disruptive behavior, while in the depressed phase they may need to encourage activity or even assist the young person in basic activities of daily living such as self-care. Similarly, clinicians may find themselves also having an impact on the young person's independence by involuntarily admitting them to hospital, enforcing medication adherence, or setting behavioral limits.

Characteristics of young people with bipolar disorder

While early studies reported no differences in presentation or outcome between early- and late-onset bipolar disorder (reviewed in Leboyer et al., 2005), this has recently been significantly challenged. Bipolar disorder that first presents at a young age is associated with a number of negative outcome variables, including:

Poor insight
A recent large study found that less than 35% of young people with affective psychosis had insight during first contact with services (Conus et al., 2007). Clearly this has significant implications, perhaps most notably that young people may be less likely to seek or accept help and may fail to engage with mental health services due to not believing there is a problem.

Symptom severity

In the Oregon Adolescent Depression Project, Lewinsohn et al. (2003) reported that of their population (whose mean age at baseline was 16.6 years), "over half of the bipolar disorder adolescents exhibited a chronic/recurrent course" (p. 49), with 12% having unremitted symptoms at age 24. The young people with mania at EPPIC obtained mean initial Global Assessment of Functioning (GAF) (American Psychiatric Association, 1994) scores of 28.7 (sd 8.5) at intake, which indicates extremely low functioning, and had mean Young Mania Rating Scale (Young et al., 1978) scores of 36.7 (sd 7.2) (Hasty et al., 2006), where a score of 20 or above is seen as meeting caseness for a manic episode.

Comorbidity

Higher comorbidity with most Axis I disorders, including substance abuse, has been identified in the early-onset population (Perlis et al., 2004).

- A review by Conus and McGorry (2002) found *significant* alcohol use in 24–39% of young people with first-episode bipolar disorder, and this was associated with poorer initial outcome, delayed onset of recovery, and shorter remission times. Similarly, a number of researchers including Ernst and Goldberg (2004) have found high rates of substance use (16–35%) in a young bipolar population. In the EPPIC bipolar population, 69% of the young people assessed had used cannabis in the 3 months prior to seeking treatment (Hasty et al., 2006). This is significant, as Tohen et al. (2000) found drug abuse or dependence was associated with poorer psychosocial outcome and lower probability of recovery at 2 years. Of additional concern is that substance abuse in adolescents can result in a 2.6-fold increase in dropout from treatment (Graf-Schimmelmann et al., 2006).
- People with early-onset bipolar disorder have also been found to present with more psychotic symptoms (Tohen et al., 1990; Carlson et al., 2000; Perlis et al., 2004).

Medication adherence

Young people with bipolar disorder have been found to have poorer medication adherence than older people with the disorder (Jamison & Akiskal, 1983; Tacchi & Scott, 2005). This is problematic, as adolescents appear to experience more rapid relapse than adults when they prematurely stop taking their medication. For example, a naturalistic study by Strober et al. (1990) found that 92% of adolescents who discontinued medication against medical advice had relapsed by 18 months, compared to 37% of completers. These rates of relapse appear considerably higher than reported in most adult studies.

Suicidal behavior

Suicidal behavior and self-harm have been found to be more common in people with early-onset, compared to later-onset, bipolar disorder (Perlis et al., 2004; Leboyer et al., 2005). This may be at least partly related to research indicating that people with pediatric-onset bipolar disorder are more likely to experience mixed states, which are associated with a higher incidence of suicidal behavior (Pavuluri et al., 2004).

Time to recovery and relapse

Carlson et al. (2000) found that people with bipolar disorder who experienced their first episode before the age of 21 had significantly longer inpatient admissions than people with adult onset (i.e. first episode after the age of 30) (a mean duration of 6.8 weeks compared with 3.7 weeks).

Young people with bipolar disorder are significantly more likely to have had a manic relapse at 24 months, compared with people with adult onset. People who have their first episode before age 21 are also less likely to remit at 24 months than those who experienced their first episode after age 30 (Carlson et al., 2000).

Psychosocial and functional outcome
Functional outcome is often poor in bipolar disorder in general, with Tohen et al. (2000) reporting that while 97% of people met criteria for syndromal recovery at 24 months, only 38% achieved functional recovery (based on residential and occupational status).

Considerable evidence indicates that functional recovery is even worse for people whose first episode occurs during adolescence. For example, Strakowski et al. (2000) found that people developing bipolar disorder prior to age 20 were significantly less likely (44% versus 62%) to achieve recovery across 4 areas of functioning at 8-month follow-up. While the younger-onset group fared more poorly across all 4 areas of recovery (role performance, interpersonal relationships, sexual activity, and recreational enjoyment), role performance was particularly impaired in this group. Similarly, Lish et al. (1994) found that people who first experienced bipolar symptoms in childhood or adolescence reported higher rates of unemployment, school dropout, substance use, financial difficulties, petty crime, self-harm, and relationship difficulties.

As functional outcome is correlated with premorbid employment status (Strakowski et al., 1998), it is understandable that young people with no secure training or employment history have poorer outcomes than those who develop the disorder later. As Tohen et al. (2000) noted, somewhat worryingly, "when functional recovery was not achieved early, it was rarely attained later" (p. 226).

Recently, the literature has presented a fairly pessimistic view of early-onset bipolar disorder, with a review (Leboyer et al., 2005) summarizing it thus: "Early onset (is) associated with greater severity and poorer long-term outcome, as shown by the chronic nature of the disorder, its resistance to mood stabilizers and the high levels of comorbidity" (p. 113).

Opportunities for early psychological intervention following a first episode

Despite the challenging characteristics of an earlier-onset bipolar population noted above, it appears likely that, as with untreated psychosis, reducing the duration of untreated mania may impact positively on the likelihood of relapse and outcome (Conus & McGorry, 2002). Utilizing a structured psychological intervention, early intervention can also offer the following opportunities:

- Early intervention may prevent suicide. The mean length of time between onset of bipolar disorder and receiving maintenance treatment has been estimated as 8.38 years, with most (73.5%) first life-threatening suicide attempts occurring within this latency period (Baldessarini et al., 1999). In their large 34–8 year prospective follow-up study, Angst et al. (2002) noted that people who developed a major mood disorder around the age of 20 presented with a significantly increased risk of suicide. However, Angst and colleagues also found that for people with bipolar I disorder, treatment significantly reduced the risk of suicide, with 6.1% of those who were treated committing suicide versus 17% who were untreated. They noted that this difference was more marked for bipolar disorder than for unipolar depression, clearly indicating the importance and effectiveness of early intervention for this population.

- Although there are reports to the contrary (e.g. Coryell et al., 1998), some research indicates that medication effectiveness, and particularly that of lithium, may be reduced with successive episodes (Gelenberg et al., 1989; Swann et al., 1999). Therefore working to improve medication adherence at first presentation may be the best opportunity for effective biological treatment.

- Psychological intervention may also be more effective early in the course of the disorder. As mentioned earlier, Scott et al. (2006) found that people with less than 12 episodes obtained better outcomes with CBT, with a "dose effect" suggesting that CBT became less effective with each episode. While Lam (2006) suggested that this *post hoc* observation should be viewed cautiously as it was not a primary hypothesis, it remains an interesting finding with notable clinical implications.

- There is evidence that with longer duration of the disorder, episodes occur more closely together with shorter periods of inter-episode wellness (Zis et al., 1980; Roy-Byrne et al., 1985; Kessing, 1998), again highlighting the importance of early intervention to prevent relapse. In animal studies, Post et al. (1986) found that progressively less and less electric current was required in order to induce seizures, to the point that eventually seizures would occur with no shock being required. Post and colleagues suggested that there may be a similar process in people with bipolar disorder, namely that with each episode, it takes progressively less stimulation or stress to precipitate a relapse. This "kindling" hypothesis has been controversial, with a large study by Kessing et al. (2004) failing to find evidence for either increased susceptibility to stressful events, or for "immunization" against them in humans. However, anecdotally some young people appear to become more vulnerable to relapse with what appear both objectively and subjectively to be decreasing levels of psychosocial stress immediately prior to each episode.

- Early intervention may help prevent secondary morbidity, as multiple episodes are associated with financial difficulties, employment difficulties, and self-esteem, guilt, loss, and adjustment issues (Scott, 1995).

- As people with bipolar disorder who experience multiple episodes can have high rates of disrupted relationships (Coryell et al., 1985), early intervention allows for work with families or partners to prevent deterioration or breakdown of relationships.

- Intervention during the early phase provides the opportunity for accurate early psychoeducation, encouragement of hope, and reduction of distress for individuals with bipolar disorder and their families.

The need for psychological treatment specific to first-episode bipolar disorder

Whilst a number of excellent psychosocial treatment manuals for bipolar disorder exist (see Introduction in this manual), it appears that there are a number of issues relevant to working with a young population that is early in the course of the disorder, which are not comprehensively covered in the existing literature. These include:

- Acknowledging the importance of engaging people with first-episode bipolar disorder in treatment, and developing interventions to assist with this.
- Awareness of the person's developmental stage and the impact of this on symptoms, course, and treatment of the disorder. The clinician should be particularly aware of the impact of the disorder on the person's psychosocial development.
- Assisting with medication adherence, which is noted to be particularly poor in this population.
- Working with people on the impact of the disorder on their developing sense of self.
- Encouraging the development of insight in a way that avoids the risk of the person rejecting potentially helpful treatment, or prevents the person from catastrophizing or overidentifying with the disorder, which is perhaps equally destructive.
- Encouraging relapse-prevention work, particularly given the high statistical likelihood of relapse, even during the first 18 months of treatment (Gitlin et al., 1995).
- Involvement of family members, given considerations relating to the developmental stage of the young person and the systemic nature of the disorder.
- Emphasizing functional recovery.

EPPIC psychological intervention for first-episode bipolar disorder

The EPPIC psychological intervention is based on individual formulation, drawing from eight key modules, which address a number of the most significant issues affecting young people with bipolar disorder. A formulation-based approach is encouraged rather than a standardized "session-by-session" intervention due to awareness that bipolar disorder may require phase-specific interventions (Swartz & Frank, 2001), and increasing recognition that individual formulation-based treatments may be more flexible and clinically useful than interventions based on diagnostic categories (British Psychological Society, 2000; Persons, 2006).

It should also be noted that the EPPIC programme provides a service for young people for up to two years, and that this manual describes an intervention that can be conducted over this period of time. In this respect it may differ from some traditionally described interventions that report around 24 sessions. However, while key aspects of the intervention can be drawn from and included in a briefer intervention, work with this population including meaningful engagement, attending to underlying schemas, adaptation to the disorder, work with families, assisting functional recovery, and management of potential relapse may often require longer-term work.

The effectiveness of the intervention will be largely dependent on the clinician's awareness of the specific difficulties and strengths experienced by the young person, the phase of the disorder and recovery, and on introducing each part of the intervention in an individualistic way in respect of this. While the effectiveness of this model is clearly challenging to assess empirically as a result of this flexibility, the heterogeneity of people with bipolar disorder demands an intervention that is adapted uniquely for each person.

Figure 1.2 illustrates the modules of intervention, with each being described in a corresponding chapter.

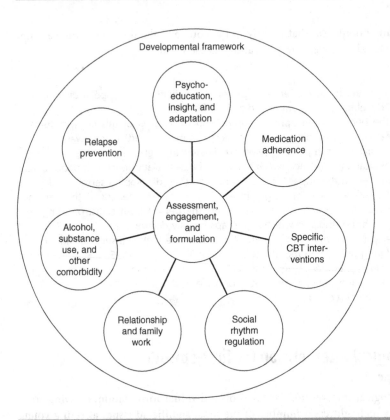

Figure 1.2 Modules of psychological intervention.

Conclusions

- Bipolar disorder has the potential to be chronic, recurrent, and traumatic for young people and their families.
- While biological and genetic factors clearly play a significant part in its etiology, and mood stabilizers appear to remain a fundamental part of treatment, medication does not appear to meet the broad spectrum of needs of many people with bipolar disorder.
- A dominant etiological model that adequately explains bipolar disorder has yet to be established, and it may be that the disorder is too complex and heterogeneous to be defined within any single model, whether biological or psychosocial. However, a number of existing models identify psychological processes that can help clinicians understand and modify symptomatology and risk of relapse.
- Recent psychological models suggest that attributional style, life events, and their impact on social rhythm may have a significant role in the development of bipolar disorder and likelihood of relapse.
- The first episode provides some specific challenges but is also a unique opportunity for effective psychosocial intervention.
- Existing psychological interventions appear to require modification to be applicable to a young, first-episode bipolar population, and should involve a strong awareness of the impact of developmental issues.
- Key issues in work with young people with bipolar disorder include developing engagement and a good treatment alliance, maintaining an awareness of the young person's developmental stage, preventing secondary morbidity, involvement of significant others in the treatment process, and finding ways of discussing the disorder which do not minimize or create undue anxiety about its course and potential outcome.

2 Assessment and engagement

The core of all treatments, biological and psychosocial, lies in the clinical relationship which develops between patients and professionals.

McGlashan et al. (1990, p. 182)

Diagnostic difficulties in bipolar disorder

There is growing acknowledgement that bipolar disorder may be significantly under-diagnosed (Bowden, 2001). For example, Hirschfeld and colleagues' (2003) survey of over 600 members of the US National Depressive and Manic Depressive Association (now known as the Depression and Bipolar Support Alliance) found that 69% of people with bipolar disorder reported having been misdiagnosed at least once. Furthermore, over one-third of respondents had a latency period of at least 10 years between initially seeking help and receiving the correct diagnosis and treatment. Unfortunately there was little change in rates of misdiagnosis between this survey, in 2003, and when it was previously conducted in 1994.

Underdiagnosis and misdiagnosis in bipolar disorder result in part from its complexity and overlap of symptoms with other disorders. Unipolar depression appears to be the most common misdiagnosis, which is understandable as many individuals have 2 or 3 depressive episodes before they experience the first manic or hypomanic episode. Ghaemi et al. (2000a) reported that around 40% of people with bipolar disorder are initially misdiagnosed with unipolar depression, while Angst (2006) suggested that, using the broadest available criteria, between one-quarter and half of people diagnosed with unipolar depression may in fact meet the criteria for bipolar disorder. This is of some concern given that diagnosis of unipolar depression may lead to the prescription of antidepressants, which some research suggests increase the risk of "switching" into mania or hypomania (Bowden, 2001).

There are a number of reasons why a person with bipolar disorder may be misdiagnosed with unipolar depression, including:

- The index episode of bipolar disorder is typically depression.
- People tend to spend over three times as much time experiencing depressive symptoms compared with manic symptoms (Judd et al., 2002), and are therefore more likely to present to a clinician as depressed.
- Primary care physicians are the professionals who are most likely to diagnose people with initial symptoms of bipolar disorder. However, the disorder can be difficult to detect in a single or even small number of brief clinical interviews.
- People are more likely to spontaneously report depressive symptoms to health professionals (Ghaemi et al., 2002) as they are distressing, and clinicians may be more likely to inquire about these. Conversely, people may be unlikely to seek treatment for mild manic symptoms that may not be noted or problematic.
- The DSM-IV-TR (American Psychiatric Association, 2000) is one of the most commonly used diagnostic guides in psychiatry. However, its criteria for bipolar

disorder may be too restrictive (i.e. manic symptoms need to have been present for at least 7 days), and the diagnosis for unipolar depression may be overly liberal.

Carlson (1985) and others have suggested that clinicians have traditionally been especially reluctant to diagnose bipolar disorder in young people. A review by McElroy et al. (1997) supported this, referencing multiple papers that identified underdiagnosis of bipolar disorder in children and adolescents. However, it is perhaps not surprising that there may be more confusion and controversy regarding diagnosis of bipolar disorder in young people, with additional complexity in this population due to mood fluctuation and substance use being common in adolescence.

Kestenbaum (1982) found that 20% of 60 young adolescents in their prospective study who were given an initial diagnosis of unipolar depression were rediagnosed with bipolar disorder within the 4-year follow-up. Kestenbaum suggested that factors which differentiated people who went on to develop bipolar disorder were: "1) rapid symptom onset, psychomotor retardation, and mood congruent psychotic features; 2) strongly positive family history of affective disorder (often bipolar); and 3) pharmacologically induced hypomania" (p. 251). Similarly, Bowden (2001) suggested that an earlier age of onset of depressive symptoms, more rapid symptom onset, and a greater amount of time spent unwell were indicative of bipolar disorder rather than major depression.

While unipolar depression remains the most common misdiagnosis, there is also evidence that adolescents with bipolar disorder are misdiagnosed with psychotic spectrum disorders, adjustment disorder (Carlson, 1985), or Axis II disorders (Morriss, 2002) including narcissistic, antisocial, and borderline personality disorder, especially where there is comorbid substance use. The most common early manifestations of overarousal and anxiety disorders are also frequently diagnosed before the presence of more typical bipolar symptoms are identified. Adolescents may also be more likely than adults to present with insidious rather than acute onset, which may make it harder to detect and contribute to delayed treatment.

In children, the diagnosis of bipolar disorder differs between continents and there is considerable debate about the differential diagnosis of childhood-onset bipolar disorder and attention deficit hyperactivity disorder and/or their co-occurrence, and the overlap between bipolar disorder and oppositional defiant and/or conduct disorders (Pavuluri et al., 2004). Advocates of childhood onset suggest that bipolar symptoms may present differently (Biederman et al., 2001). Specifically, young people appear more likely than adults to present with mixed states (26% versus 3%) (Carlson et al., 2000) or depressive symptoms, and irritability may be more common than euphoria in young adolescents (Pavuluri et al., 2004; Biederman et al., 2005). The subject remains controversial, not least because of concerns regarding the prescription of long-term mood stabilizers in children.

Psychological assessment: a case formulation approach

The effectiveness of any treatment programme, pharmacological or psychological, depends on its ability to target selective problems in specific phases of the illness.

Lam (2006, p. 321)

Although a number of CBT manuals describe standardized interventions, and at times even session-by-session plans, it is essential that psychological treatment is not simply a mechanical, standardized process. As Erickson and Rossi (1979) noted, "each psychotherapeutic encounter is unique and requires fresh creative effort on the part of both the therapist and patient to discover the principles and means of achieving a therapeutic outcome" (p. 234).

It is clear that therapists are not simply vehicles to deliver techniques, and instead that the selection of the right technique at the right time, the relationship between the therapist and the client, and a shared understanding of the goals and how these will be achieved are critical aspects of the process (Scott & Colom, 2008).

Bipolar disorder can be extremely complex, and people with this diagnosis are unique in their personal histories, etiologies, symptoms, levels of impairment, and strengths. To assume a "one size fits all" approach, particularly with a young bipolar population, may be at best naive, and at worst ineffective and potentially harmful. For example, insisting on providing extensive standardized psychoeducation regarding bipolar disorder to some-one who is ambivalent or unwilling to accept their diagnosis may cause a young person to become distressed, disengage from therapy, or even feel suicidal (see Chapter 3 for further details). The initial focus is the therapeutic relationship, and the pace (unless significant risk factors are present) will be dictated by the young person's ability to discuss and adapt to their new circumstances. The initial discussion often focuses on uncovering the details of what has happened to bring the individual to the attention of the services.

Initially, a thorough assessment of presenting symptoms should be undertaken. This should be followed by inquiry about previous and current personal, family, social, and occupational functioning, while also screening for comorbid disorders, identifying associ-ated secondary morbidity, and considering differential diagnoses. Following this, the clinician should develop a formulation, incorporating the person's history, premorbid functioning, and predisposing, precipitating, perpetuating, prognostic, and protective factors, in addition to considering individual treatment goals for the specific phase of the disorder. This is important because of the heterogeneity of people with bipolar disorder, and due to the fact that there can be four different mood presentations when a person is symptomatic (manic, hypomanic, depressed, and mixed), each of which requires a different clinical approach.

As our intervention utilizes a largely CBT approach, psychological assessment and the development of an individualized CBT formulation are undertaken (see Chapter 5 and Figure 5.3). This involves identifying the contribution of early developmental and attach-ment history, family factors, and critical life events to the evolution of particular automatic thoughts, schemas, and behavioral patterns that could be related to the disorder for that person. For example, in his work on depression, Gilbert (2000) noted how early experience, such as neglect or criticism, can shape a young person's beliefs, particularly regarding how they view themselves and the world, and may lead to behavior such as avoidance, which in turn could then maintain these beliefs. Similarly, in their development of schema therapy, Young et al. (2003) described the importance of early life events and how "toxic childhood experiences" (p. 10) can shape unhelpful and persistent thinking patterns and behavior.

Clinical assessment

(1) Symptomatology and previous treatment

This involves identifying key aspects of the person's current presentation, including a thorough investigation of all the person's symptoms, comorbidities, and contextual or environmental factors relating to onset and maintenance of symptoms. Assessment should also include a thorough historical investigation of previous symptoms, including whether the young person has experienced clinical or subclinical depressive, manic, or hypomanic symptoms in addi-tion to the existence of symptoms of other disorders, particularly anxiety. If treatment was received for any of these, the young person and their family should be asked about their experience of this, and their understanding of these symptoms.

(2) Biological assessment

Before providing a psychological intervention, it is essential that a thorough physical assessment has been undertaken to rule out symptoms which may be secondary to illicit substance use (particularly amphetamines and hallucinogens), head injury, tumors, infections (including influenza), or other illnesses including hyperthyroidism and vitamin B-12 deficiency (Torrey & Knable, 2002). Assessment could include CT or MRI scan, EEG, routine blood tests (full blood examination, liver function tests, thyroid function tests), tests for HIV and hepatitis, and urine drug screens (EPPIC, unpublished document), contingent on clinical indication and resource availability. It is also important to assess use of prescription medications that have been associated with the onset of manic symptoms, including anabolic steroids and corticosteroids, benzodiazepines, disulfiram (Antabuse®), some antidepressants including monoamine oxidase inhibitors (MAOIs) and selective serotonin reuptake inhibitors (SSRIs), and methylphenidate (Ritalin®) (Torrey & Knable, 2002).

Biological assessment should also ensure that any medical or physical health needs are met.

(3) Personal history

This includes assessing relevant attachment history, significant developmental incidents, and premorbid functioning and personality. The clinician should inquire about the following areas and their impact:

- Birth order or role; for example, the responsibility of looking after younger siblings or expectations which may result following the success of an elder sibling.
- Care and quality of relationships with family and significant others.
- Medical history and previous involvement of the young person or family member with health services, particularly mental health services.
- Physical development including onset of puberty.
- Traumatic experiences including physical, sexual, or emotional abuse.
- Deaths or loss of significant others, the person's individual response to this, and how this was managed within the family.
- Separations from significant others.
- Religious, social, or political beliefs within the family.
- Illness or hospitalizations of self or significant others.
- Rewards and punishments within the family.
- Criticism, overinvolvement, and placement of guilt.
- Geographical moves.
- Relationship breakdown, including separation or divorce of parents.
- Social functioning, including relationships with friends and, if appropriate, sexual relationships.
- School performance or work history.
- Legal or forensic history.
- Strengths, successes, and achievements.

Part of this can also include asking the young person what "messages" they grew up with, and what they thought were the key issues their parents or significant others passed on to them about themselves, the world, and the future.

(4) Family history

There is growing research on the influence of bonding and attachment and its impact on mental health, with evidence that attachment difficulties can impact on a number of mental health disorders, including depression (Mason et al., 2005). A large study by Heider et al. (2006)

utilized the Parental Bonding Inventory (PBI) with over 8000 participants across 6 European countries. They identified a clear and consistent correlation between perceived lack of parental care and increased occurrence of mood disorders by around 20%. While recognizing the PBI is a retrospective measure, these findings are consistent with the majority of research in this area. In a later study, Heider et al. (2007) found a significant correlation between reported lack of parental care and suicidality, even when controlling for lifetime mood or anxiety disorders, and lifetime alcohol abuse or dependence.

Diamond and Doane (1994) suggested: "Internal working models of attachment hold a central place in adolescents and adults" (p. 778). They also noted: "There is increasing evidence that such internal working models of attachment are stable and enduring, not only within the individual over time . . . but also within families across generations" (p. 771). Clearly therefore, assessing family factors, including structure, roles, relationships between individuals, and attachment issues, can be useful. Identifying unhelpful interactive patterns can be a particularly important focus of assessment and may have significant implications for treatment.

Constructing a genogram of relationships between family members can also be valuable, and McGoldrick et al. (2008) provide a detailed description of assessment and clinical implications of this. A strong understanding of each family member's explanatory model of the person's disorder can also be important, as can awareness of any health or psychiatric issues in other family members, because these may have significant implications for the young person's own explanatory model and preconceptions around the disorder and treatment. Further details are in Chapter 7.

(5) Risk issues
The clinician should assess the young person for risk of self-harm or suicide, vulnerability, neglect (including self-neglect), and the likelihood of harming others, particularly due to impulsivity.

(6) Alcohol and substance use
Past or current illicit substance and alcohol use should be assessed given the particularly high prevalence of these in the bipolar population. Further details regarding assessment of, and interventions for, this are described in Chapter 8.

(7) Motivation and insight
Motivation regarding treatment and insight, including the person's explanatory model of their current experiences, should be assessed. Typically, this would include asking open, non-pathologizing questions such as:
- "Why do you come along to this center?"
- "Why did you go to hospital?"
- "Why are you taking medicine?/Why are people asking you to take medication at the moment?"
- "What have people said about what they think is happening for you at the moment? Do you agree with them?"

This is discussed further in Chapter 3.

(8) Assessment of schemas
Schemas have been defined as "core beliefs which . . . play a central role in the maintenance of long-term psychiatric problems" (Padesky, 1994, p. 267). Schemas are seen as ways in which people attend to, group, and process information, and in cognitive therapy are seen as relating to three main areas: how the person views themselves, how they view others, and how they view the world (Beck et al., 1979).

Understanding schemas of people with bipolar disorder is important, as they can give an insight into the way a person views the world, and how they may feel and behave in response to particular experiences. The Young Schema Questionnaire (YSQ-L3) (Young & Brown, 2005) can be a useful assessment tool, as it gives insight into the person's beliefs across different domains, including beliefs about personal competence, approval-seeking, or vulnerability. It also allows for discussion about schemas that are unhelpful or contribute to current symptomatology or risk of relapse. The use of the YSQ-L3 as a therapeutic tool will be discussed in more detail in Chapter 5.

Taking such an interest and clearly trying to understand the person's inner experiences of the world comprises an essential part of the engagement process.

Engagement and the therapeutic alliance

The therapeutic relationship has been found to be crucially important in a number of therapy approaches, and can impact significantly on clinical outcomes in a number of disorders (Teyber & McClure, 2000). Keijsers et al. (2000) suggested that the therapeutic relationship accounts for 5–20% of the outcome variance, while Crits-Cristoph et al. (1991) found that the therapeutic alliance accounted for a higher variance in outcome (21%) than treatment models including CBT, interpersonal therapy, and placebo pharmacotherapy.

Regarding specific disorders, Frank and Gunderson (1990) found that people diagnosed with schizophrenia who were rated by their clinicians as having good therapeutic alliance were less likely to drop out of treatment, had better medication adherence, and had better functional outcomes. The same appears true for mood disorders, with Blatt et al. (1996) having studied therapist characteristics in a large US National Institute of Mental Health (NIMH) sponsored study on depression, the Treatment of Depression Collaborative Research Program (TDCRP). Blatt and colleagues stated: "Therapeutic gain in the TDCRP is significantly influenced by interpersonal dimensions of the treatment process – by patient and therapist capacity to establish a therapeutic relationship" (p. 1277).

The therapeutic alliance, as measured by the Working Alliance Inventory (Horvath & Greenberg, 1989) and the California Psychotherapy Alliance Scale (Gaston, 1991), has been found to be a reliable indicator of outcome in depression and affective disorders, with better therapeutic relationships being correlated with better clinical outcomes and reduced likelihood of dropout (Keijsers et al., 2000). For bipolar disorder specifically, patients who were more satisfied with their clinicians were found to adapt better to their diagnosis, cope better with the disorder, and report feeling less ashamed or angry, than those who were less satisfied with their clinicians (Hirschfeld et al., 2003).

While there is recognition that engagement and a strong therapeutic relationship are essential, establishing these can be difficult, given that even for CBT – a model widely recognized as collaborative and effective – premature dropout rates have been estimated at around 40% (Leahy, 2001). Furthermore, even in a specialized early psychosis service, rates of around 28% premature treatment dropout have been reported (Graf-Schimmelmann et al., 2006).

Graf-Schimmelmann et al. (2006) found that the two most significant predictors of dropout for young people with psychotic disorders (including bipolar disorder with psychotic features) were persistent illicit substance use during the treatment period (resulting in a 2.6-fold increased likelihood of premature termination of therapy) and lack of family support (leading to a 4.8-fold increased likelihood of dropout). Interestingly, they found neither insight at baseline nor substance use at baseline were predictive of premature dropout from treatment. In contrast, people who remain in therapy have expressed confidence in their therapists' skills, agreed with what was being planned as well as how targets would be addressed, and noted that their clinicians appeared to respect them and their viewpoints (Davidson & Scott, 2008).

The therapeutic relationship in bipolar disorder

Difficulties in engagement and establishing a therapeutic relationship, which can be encountered in any therapy, are often compounded when working with people with bipolar disorder. This is because manic or hypomanic symptoms may not be of concern to the person experiencing them, and may in fact be a welcome respite for people who have previously had lengthy episodes of depression or dysthymia. Furthermore, individuals with bipolar disorder are often more interpersonally demanding than individuals with disorders that are less likely to produce periods of activation (Scott, 2003).

> **Case study 2.1: Alexander**
>
> Alexander, an 18-year-old man with bipolar disorder, reported: "Mania is the most amazing experience a person could have. You can take delight in the smallest thing, and simultaneously think about the biggest things. It feels like there's nothing you can't do. Well not much anyway. The only downside is that you don't understand why people around you are sad."

Clearly in the case study above, there appeared little incentive for Alexander to engage in treatment and be "cured" of his manic symptoms. Kahn (1990) acknowledged this difficulty, stating that "mania turns the therapeutic relationship upside down," and added that mania is a disorder "that a patient finds so pleasurable and a psychiatrist so frustrating that neither feels any zeal for talking to the other" (p. 230). Therefore, as opposed to most other disorders in which all parties are seeking symptom resolution, the goals of the person with bipolar disorder and the clinician may initially appear to differ markedly, particularly in the manic or hypomanic phase.

In addition to the engagement challenges facing people with bipolar disorder themselves, Goodwin and Jamison (1990) acknowledged issues that may face therapists working with this population, and the importance of counter-transference in bipolar disorder. Specifically, they noted that fluctuating mood, irritability, aggression, denial, disinhibition, and "tuning in to the therapist's jugular" (p. 734) – which may occur when a person is hypomanic – or suicide attempts and hopelessness when a person is depressed, can lead to anger, impotence, and feelings of failure on the part of the therapist. Bateman et al. (1954) also noted some of the challenges presented by people when manic. They stated: "The listener becomes fatigued by the constant diversions and shifts in the sequence of thought, which is complicated by diffuse detail and yet completely restricted to a narrow range of personal references and preoccupations. Inevitably, the patient reveals an unabashedly self-centred, unadaptive, aggressive and superior attitude, even though he sometimes makes an attempt to be friendly and cooperative" (p. 350).

Issues relating to control have been identified as particularly important in the therapeutic relationship when working with bipolar disorder. Goodwin and Jamison (1990) acknowledged this in the following quote from a patient with bipolar disorder: "The endless questioning finally ended. My psychiatrist looked at me, there was no uncertainty in his voice. 'Manic depressive illness.' I admired his bluntness. I wished him locusts on his lands and a pox upon his house. Silent, unbelievable rage. I smiled pleasantly. He smiled back. The war had just begun" (p. 746).

Dooley (1921) described a similarly combative relationship, stating: "Those who manifest frequent manic attacks are likely to be headstrong, self-sufficient, know-it-all types of persons who will not take suggestion or yield to direction. They are 'doers' and managers, and will get the upper hand of the analyst and everyone else around them if given an opportunity" (p. 39). Dooley later stated: "The transference seems good but the analyst is really only an appendage to the greatly inflated ego" (p. 39). While this is not the case for the majority of young people we see, it nonetheless illustrates the frustration experienced by some clinicians working with this population.

Goodwin and Jamison (2007) advised therapists on managing these issues, stating: "The psychotherapy of bipolar disorder requires considerable flexibility in style and technique. Flexibility is necessary because of the patient's changing mood, thinking, and behavior as well as the fluctuating levels of therapeutic dependency intrinsic to the illness . . . A thin line exists between too much and too little therapeutic control: too much may lead to increased dependency, maladaptive rebellion, decreased self-esteem, or non-adherence; too little may lead to feelings of insecurity, an unnecessarily tenuous hold on reality, and feelings of abandonment" (p. 872). This may be of increased importance when working with young people, as issues of control and independence may be even more marked, and mishandling these may exacerbate an already potentially tenuous therapeutic alliance.

Engagement can also be particularly difficult early in the course of bipolar disorder, given that symptoms may not yet have become as destructive to functioning and relationships as for people with a longer history of the disorder. Furthermore, in a young population in which people have often not experienced any significant health difficulties, let alone mental health difficulties, and may have only been experiencing symptoms for a very short period of time, it can be challenging to engage and help a person understand that long-term work may be required.

A final challenge in working with bipolar disorder is that of the "seduction" of mania and hypomania. An empathic therapist who is keen to develop a good therapeutic relationship may need to guard against unconsciously mirroring and colluding with a young person experiencing a manic or hypomanic episode.

However, it is important to note that a good therapeutic relationship may be formed even when the person's mood is unstable, with Kahn (1990) suggesting "there is value in talking with bipolar patients, even while they are manic, not only about the need to take medication, but also about themselves and their experience of illness" (p. 229).

Characteristics of a positive therapeutic relationship
Therapist factors

A recent comprehensive review of the impact of therapist factors on the therapeutic relationship (Ackerman & Hilsenroth, 2003) identified a number of attributes and techniques associated with a positive therapeutic alliance. This included elements defined in the client-centered psychotherapy literature (Rogers, 1976) such as the therapist's expression of accurate empathy, and their ability to express themselves clearly, to connect with the person, to be flexible, warm, genuine, respectful, friendly, trustworthy, interested, alert, competent, and to work collaboratively. Techniques identified as helpful, regardless of psychotherapeutic model, included exploration, depth, identifying past successes, accurate interpretation, being active in therapy, and acknowledging the person's experience.

Notably, a recent review found that when asked their preferences regarding treatment, around two-thirds of people with bipolar disorder said they would like their psychiatrists to "listen better" (Lewis, 2005). Of concern is that many people stated that they would not report symptoms to their clinicians, and while 69% of their sample had thoughts of death or had considered suicide, only 49% reported this to their doctors.

Client factors

While much of the research has focused on therapist factors that help establish a positive therapeutic relationship, it should be noted that the therapeutic relationship is bidirectional, and that the client is also able to generate warmth, trust, respect, and openness. As Sullivan et al. (2005) noted on therapy outcome, perhaps with no small measure of sarcasm, "although the most important pantheoretical variable appears to be the client . . . the therapist is another promising variable" (p. 48).

Specifically, the client's openness to describing their difficulties and disclosing personal information has been identified as related to treatment outcome (Keijsers et al., 2000). However, while self-exploration and insight are described as key elements of psychoanalytic and client-centered therapy, Orlinsky and Howard's (1986) review found a non-significant correlation between these factors and outcome in 26 of 36 studies. This would suggest that while it is important for people to understand their difficulties, this may not be enough to facilitate a positive clinical outcome.

Finally, Keijsers et al. (2000) found a significant relationship between expressed motivation by clients and clinical outcome in 13 of 18 empirical studies. This may relate to patients' expectations and hope, which have been recognized as playing powerful roles in outcome (Meyer et al., 2002), with Weinberger and Eig (1999) describing patient expectancy as "the ignored common factor in psychotherapy" (p. 357).

Engagement and establishing a positive therapeutic relationship in young people with bipolar disorder

The following may assist the clinician in developing good therapeutic relationships with young people in the early phase of bipolar disorder:

Not assuming "psychological mindedness" or "motivation." We find that, specifically when working with young people with bipolar disorder, "psychological mindedness" is the exception rather than the rule, and is therefore not a prerequisite for psychological intervention. When working with this population, we feel strongly that it is the responsibility of the clinician to collaboratively support the development of psychological mindedness, and that motivation can emerge in the context of a good therapeutic relationship.

Involvement with the person from initial onset of the disorder. Practically, this may involve meeting the person at an inpatient unit during the acute phase, even if this only involves very brief initial introductory sessions for the clinician to describe his/her role. This can be particularly valuable not only for engagement, but later in therapy when the therapist's ability to identify idiosyncratic symptoms may assist the recognition and prevention of potential relapse.

Continuity of care. While real world considerations may interfere with this, we have found engagement is assisted by having a regular clinician. This avoids the inconvenience for the young person of having to re-tell their history numerous times, and allows him/her and family members to have a consistent point of contact. A regular clinician may also be more likely to identify subtle mood or behavioral changes that may be missed by someone who has had less contact with the young person.

Awareness of the young person's requirements at their particular stage of recovery. Maslow's (1943) hierarchy of needs can serve as a useful model in this respect. Maslow suggested that people have a number of motivations that can be organized in a hierarchy from the basic to the more complex. These include physiological needs (including water, food, and reasonable temperature), safety needs (including emotional support, routine, and protection from harm), and esteem and self-actualization, which involve attaining confidence and independence, undertaking activities which the person feels they are "meant for," understanding the world, and feeling understood. When working with young people with bipolar disorder, the clinician may need to focus on a hierarchical intervention incorporating issues such as:

- Attending to immediate physical health concerns.
- Ensuring stable and safe accommodation.
- Offering assistance with financial issues (including accumulated debts).
- Assisting with legal issues (including legal charges which may be related to behavior when manic).
- Enhancing medication adherence and screening for side-effects.
- Introducing behavioral interventions (including increasing activity in the depressive phase and reducing stimulation in the manic phase).
- Attending to substance abuse issues.
- Undertaking collaborative psychoeducation.
- Providing family work, including assisting helpful communication styles.
- Managing unhelpful automatic thoughts, including those related to the disorder.
- Helping the person adapt to the disorder.
- Schema work and behavioral interventions that may reduce the likelihood of relapse.

Assistance with practical issues. As noted above, this can be very valuable, particularly in the early phase of the therapeutic relationship. Ironically, assisting the young person with some of the aftermath of a manic episode – such as legal problems, financial difficulties, accommodation crises, and other difficulties resulting from impulsivity or disorganization – may be one of the most effective ways of establishing good engagement.

Inquiring as to the young person's previous experiences of treatment. Although young people early in the course of the disorder are unlikely to have had extensive contact with mental health professionals, it is possible that before reaching therapy they have had contact with a school counselor, primary care physician, triage or crisis team members, and possibly accident and emergency department staff. It can be particularly effective to ask about behaviors by other professionals that have either been particularly helpful or unhelpful. This demonstrates to the young person that the clinician is keen to work collaboratively, wishes to avoid making the mistakes made by other professionals, and wants to continue interventions that have been positive. Generally, young people are forthcoming about their experiences of previous treatment, and can give the clinician valuable guidance regarding what they are most likely to respond to, both positively and negatively.

Seeing the young person in their home or a "neutral" venue. While service constraints and large caseloads may limit the feasibility of this, at least during the initial stages it can help engagement and, in the case of home visits, allow the clinician to gain important additional information about the young person's environment.

The motivational interviewing literature (Miller & Rollnick, 2002) can be helpful, as can considering the young person's "stage of change" (Prochaska & DiClemente, 1986). Clearly, attempting to undertake relapse prevention work is unlikely to be effective if a person does not consider themselves as having experienced any mental health problems. This is described in more detail in Chapter 8.

Taking time to understand the person and their circumstances before providing direction or making suggestions can be important. While there are likely to be service issues which influence length of treatment, it appears important in any therapeutic relationship, and perhaps particularly with young people with bipolar disorder who may be ambivalent about treatment and keen to establish their independence, that they do not feel harassed into making changes. In his book *Overcoming Resistance in Cognitive Therapy*, Leahy (2001) quotes a person who stated of their therapist: "How can he help me if he doesn't even understand me?" (p. 2).

Openness in the therapeutic process, and explaining why particular questions are being asked, can be valuable. While the clinician may be clear as to reasons for leading the session in a particular way, the young person may not be, and it can be helpful to be transparent.

Acknowledging that change can be difficult. It is important that the clinician is aware that changing any behavior can be difficult, even when the behavior appears destructive to the person. Awareness of this can help to reduce the therapist's frustration should a person continue to abuse substances, refuse to attend appointments, or fail to take medication despite the risk of relapse.

Monitoring the dynamic in the therapeutic relationship, and being aware of the degree to which it is collaborative at any point in time, can be important. Specifically, this involves attending to the "process" rather than just the "content" of a session. Berk et al. (2004) noted that the therapeutic relationship can be at varying points on a spectrum at different stages during treatment, ranging from extremely autonomous to overly paternalistic. This can be particularly important when working with young people, where negotiating independence may be especially pertinent. For example, some young people can initially appear overly dependent and approval-seeking, which, although often ensuring medication adherence early in therapy, may not necessarily be helpful in terms of adaptation and management of the disorder.

The CBT model gives a collaborative structure to sessions and can help ensure that the young person's own agenda is being addressed. This is described in more detail in Chapter 5.

Working within the person's "zone of proximal development" (Ryle & Kerr, 2002, p. 41). This refers both to the pacing of information in sessions, and to the therapist being clear that issues are discussed at an intellectual and emotional level that the young person can comprehend.

Adapting the length of sessions to the person's stage of recovery appears important. While 45 minutes may be an optimum length for sessions when working with an adult with relatively stable mood, this may not be appropriate for a young person with attention difficulties. The clinician should be sensitive to the person's ability to tolerate the session, and retain awareness that concentration is likely to be influenced by depressive or manic symptoms.

Diagrams and visual aids can be very useful in working with young people with bipolar disorder, given that symptoms may interfere with comprehension or recall of information. For example, drawing a "bell-curve" can be an important way of highlighting the experience of mania for some young people. This identifies that while hypomania is initially often a pleasant experience, when it goes over the "crest" it is associated with irritability and frustration for many young people. This visual aid can help identify the need for treatment in an uncomplicated way.

Awareness of the person's goals at particular stages of treatment, and noting that these may differ from those of the clinician, can be important. Identifying a shared problem list appears a significant aspect of engagement, and it should be noted that goals are likely to vary depending on the phase of the disorder.

Involving family members can assist engagement. Working with family members to reinforce the importance of treatment, and to listen to and support the person, can be essential.

Understanding the young person's explanatory model. Kelly (1955) described the concept of people as "scientists" constructing their own reality, with much of cognitive therapy being based on the concept that people's construction of reality is extremely important in terms of their behavior and emotional response. Clearly, therefore, the clinician should take significant time, and have a genuine interest in the young person's understanding of what has happened to them. Scott (2001) described core questions to explore to understand the client's view:

- "What do you think it is?"
- "What do you think caused it?"
- "What have you tried to control/contain the problem – which tactics have worked/not worked?"
- "What have been the consequences of the problem so far?"
- "What do you think will happen in the future (will it recur)?"

This set of questions allows exploration of key targets for psychoeducation and puts the behavior of the individual into a "rational" framework (for example, if the young person doesn't think the problem is likely to recur, he/she would be unlikely to engage with relapse-prevention treatments).

The language used by the clinician can be particularly important in setting the tone for an intervention. Many young people do not find terms such as "bipolar disorder," "illness," or "manic depression" helpful, particularly in the early stages of engagement. Listening carefully to the language used by the young person and their own expressions can be important. For example, it may be helpful for the clinician to use similar descriptions of an episode as the young person, such as "when I skitzed out," "when I was really stressed," "when I was in hospital," "when I was really hyper," or "when things were really speedy." It is important that the clinician is careful to avoid overly medicalized or pejorative language, such as "when you were unwell/sick," "now that you have bipolar disorder," or "do you think you have a mental illness?" unless the young person has already introduced these expressions and appears comfortable with them.

Similarly, simple changes in terminology may be important (Scott, 2003), as talking about "between-session homework" may make the client feel like they are in a teacher-pupil relationship, which may be helpful to some but may provoke negative reactions in others.

Hope or optimism by the young person, their family, and the clinician appear to play a significant role in outcome, particularly in depression where it was found to be one of the best predictors of outcome (Priebe & Gruyters, 1995). As Meyer et al. (2002) noted, "patients' engagement in therapy depends on their expectations of treatment effectiveness" (p. 1051). They suggested that something of a self-fulfilling prophecy can occur, where "patients who believe that therapy can help them attain the goal of symptom reduction will work constructively at the task, and this effort tends to pay off in the future" (p. 1054). Furthermore, positive expectation may focus a patient's attention on successful aspects of therapy, with this increasing motivation and attendance. This is particularly important in engaging young people and their families, with May (2004) having noted: "Hope is a key ingredient in successful recoveries, but, traditionally this has been lacking in mental health services" (p. 249). May also emphasized that while clinicians should not create unrealistic expectations of a "cure" for significant mental health problems, they should strongly emphasize the concepts of "recovery" and gaining control over remaining difficulties.

Clinicians actually caring *about their patients.* Yalom (2002) advised therapists, "let the patient matter to you" (p. 26), and suggested further: "Learn about their (i.e. patients') lives; you will not only be edified but you will ultimately learn all you need to know about their illness"

(Yalom, 1999, p. 17). Similar to the concept of clinician hope, this may historically not have been given sufficient emphasis.

Management of ruptures or potential ruptures in the therapeutic relationship. In their review of the therapeutic alliance, Ackerman and Hilsenroth (2003) noted that "ruptures are an expected part of the treatment process" (p. 29), but that they can provide "fertile ground for patient change and an opportunity for deepening the alliance" (p. 29). Issues such as confidentiality, inpatient admission, medication adherence, independence, and management of inappropriate behavior can all be challenging to the therapeutic relationship when working with young people with bipolar disorder. It therefore appears essential that the therapist manages these successfully, and if appropriate, overtly accepts responsibility should a mistake have occurred. This is acknowledged in Sullivan et al. (2005), where an experienced therapist stated succinctly: "I still believe an apology is one of the best therapeutic tools there is" (p. 54). An interesting paper by Castonguay et al. (1996) examined the effect of therapeutic factors on outcome in CBT for depression. They found that when "therapeutic strains" (p. 501) such as avoidance of therapeutic tasks or failing to acknowledge the person's legitimate real-life concerns were not addressed directly, and the therapist instead focused more on the role of the person's cognitions or overemphasized the CBT model, the clinical outcome was poorer and depressive symptomatology increased. This may be even more notable in young people, given the potential for confrontation or ruptures resulting from poorly managed control and independence issues.

Emphasizing strengths. There is a danger that therapists become overly focused on pathology and fail to inquire about the person's strengths and achievements. As Yalom (1999) noted of a mentor who would ask his patients about their interests, "by allowing the patient to teach him, he (the therapist) related to the *person*, rather than the pathology, of that patient. His strategy invariably enhanced both the patient's self regard and his or her willingness to be self-revealing" (p. 17). Similarly, Schwartz and Flowers (2006) suggested: "It is essential that we are as methodical in our search for our clients' strengths as we are in searching for the correct clinical diagnosis" (p. 30).

Finally, the clinician should be aware that engagement is an ongoing process throughout therapy and while it is particularly important in the initial phase, it remains important even after the early sessions. Generally, ongoing vigilance and effort are required to maintain a good therapeutic relationship.

Case study 2.2: engagement and managing potential therapeutic ruptures – Sean

Sean was a 20-year-old man with recently diagnosed bipolar disorder. He had been discharged from an inpatient unit after two weeks, but remained fairly disorganized and was only able to attend when his mother drove him to appointments. The therapist had seen Sean at the inpatient unit and had a good understanding of his symptoms when manic. This helped continuity of care, as when Sean came to the outpatient department, he immediately recognized his therapist and did not have to repeat his history.

Sean had little insight, but recognized he had been "a bit racy" and had spent a lot of money impulsively. The therapist discussed with Sean what would be helpful for them to work on in future sessions. Sean wanted financial help due to a number of bills he had accumulated, and asked if the therapist could write letters to various agencies asking for delays in payment, and set up payment plans. Sean agreed to take medicine as it helped him sleep. The therapist used Sean's expressions of "racy" and "a bit wired" when discussing symptoms but did not discuss diagnosis in early sessions, as this was not deemed to be helpful at that stage, and did not appear a priority to Sean.

In generating an explanatory model, the therapist was keen to incorporate Sean's understanding as much as possible. The therapist generally took a tentative approach when making observations or expressing opinions, using expressions such as: "Sean, it seems like . . .," "I wonder if . . .," "can I check out . . .," and "it sounds like . . ." This demonstrated to Sean that the therapist was keen to understand him properly and genuinely wanted to establish a collaborative relationship. Furthermore, it illustrated to Sean that the therapist, while having knowledge of mental health issues and treatment of bipolar disorder, did not assume expertise about Sean and his unique history and experiences.

While Sean remained hypomanic, the therapist was keen to reach a balance of maintaining engagement while establishing boundaries and slowing down the pace of sessions. The therapist paid particular attention to his own rate and volume of speech, in order to give Sean a reasonably structured therapeutic environment.

Establishing boundaries was also assisted by sessions taking a reasonably standardized format. This typically consisted of beginning each session with a brief review of the previous session, setting an agenda, addressing agenda items, and summarizing at the end of each session. While it was often difficult initially to remain "on track" given Sean's disorganization, Sean did report that he felt "listened to" during his sessions.

During session 12, a significant challenge occurred to the therapeutic relationship. Although a number of his more acute manic symptoms had reduced significantly, Sean remained somewhat overfamiliar with the therapist, frequently asking mildly inappropriate and personal questions. In addition, Sean asked if the therapist would attend a social event with him, which the therapist politely explained would not be possible. This was followed by a long silence on Sean's part and then irritable and monosyllabic responses to further questions in the session. Despite the fact that Sean initially denied that his therapist declining the offer had been a problem, this had clearly upset Sean and he subsequently cancelled the following appointment. The therapist felt it was essential to address what had occurred quickly, as it appeared to be a considerable threat to their therapeutic relationship.

The therapist did this by acknowledging that refusing Sean's request may have been hurtful, and discussing possible reasons for Sean's misinterpreting the therapeutic relationship as that of a "friendship." It also raised the question of boundary issues, and gave the therapist the opportunity to explain that while keen to develop and retain a good working alliance with Sean, it was important that it remained a professional relationship. Sean was asked to describe how he felt and what he thought about the situation. Sean acknowledged that it had been hurtful to be refused, and that it had been confusing given that he thought they had a good relationship. Sean was also able to reflect that he had lost a number of his previous friends due to his symptoms, particularly his irritability and impulsiveness, but he also accepted that the relationship with his therapist should be a professional one. Sean also acknowledged that he might have been more "pushy" than normal, recognizing that he was still slightly elevated, and disclosed that he had also uncharacteristically approached a girl he did not know to ask her out.

This approach to repairing ruptures was considered important in four respects. Firstly, it allowed the opportunity to discuss the nature and boundaries of the therapeutic relationship. Secondly, it allowed for the demonstration of a collaborative model of conflict resolution, where a delicate interpersonal issue could be discussed openly, something Sean said occurred rarely within his family. Thirdly, it facilitated later discussion about how to approach people with requests for social contact, something that Sean had previously found anxiety-provoking. Finally, with some gentle humor, it was noted that the therapist had modeled "imperfect" management of this situation. This was important to Sean who had previously somewhat idealized his therapist, and had unrealistic expectations of a "perfect" therapist, which could have potentially led to later disappointment in therapy.

Time spent discussing symptoms of the disorder with Sean was balanced by a strengths-based approach, which included asking about his interests, previous functioning, and achievements. It emerged that Sean had been one of the top students in his year, had an encyclopedic knowledge of the cinema, and was a reasonable middle-distance runner. Spending some of the sessions discussing these topics assisted Sean in separating himself from his bipolar disorder, recognizing that managing his symptoms was one part, but not an all-encompassing aspect, of his life. It was also felt that this helped enhance his self-esteem and increased his motivation to attend.

Conclusions

- Bipolar disorder appears to be underdiagnosed in young people, with unipolar depression remaining the most common misdiagnosis.
- There is evidence that bipolar disorder can be accurately diagnosed in young people, but that their presentation may be different to that of adults. Most notably, young people are more likely to present with symptoms of depression and irritability during manic episodes, rather than euphoria.
- A positive therapeutic relationship has been found to be highly influential in terms of reducing the likelihood of dropping out of treatment, improving medication adherence and functional outcomes in psychotic disorders (Frank & Gunderson, 1990), and predicting better clinical outcome in mood disorders (Horvath & Greenberg, 1989).
- Engagement can be challenging with young people with bipolar disorder, as motivation for treatment may be poor, and independence issues are likely to be important. However, engagement may be one of the most crucial aspects of treatment with this population, and is arguably the foundation on which the rest of therapy is built.
- Factors which may assist engagement are: empathy, attending to the therapeutic process, continuity of care, assistance with practical issues, a strong awareness of the person's explanatory model, being respectful of the person's terminology, collaborative goal setting, and ensuring that the person's family members are supportive of the intervention.

3 Insight, adaptation, and functional recovery

That proves you mad because you know it not.

Thomas Decker (Torrey & Knable, 2002, p. 41)

In this chapter we discuss the issue of insight and ways in which young people may adapt to a diagnosis of bipolar disorder. While some young people minimize or deny their diagnosis, for others, bipolar disorder can significantly impact on their sense of self and identity, and can result in feelings of guilt, shame, loss, and trauma.

After consideration of these issues, we present strategies to help decrease distress, promote adaptive coping, and minimize the impact of the disorder on the person's view of self and their functioning. As with other chapters of this book, the strategies presented in this section are not intended to be delivered in a sequential fashion or as a discrete module. Instead, we encourage clinicians to continue to employ and revisit them where relevant throughout the intervention, recognizing that the young person's insight and needs can change across their phases of recovery and relapse.

Insight

Lack of insight has been described as a common characteristic of bipolar disorder (Pallanti et al., 1999), with some research showing that the degree of insight in bipolar disorder is similar to that of people with schizophrenia (Amador et al., 1994; Pini et al., 2001). Insight has been found to be consistently poorer for people with mania than for people with mixed episodes or unipolar depression (Dell'Osso et al., 2002). This may occur as the dysphoria and distress that happen in the depressive and mixed phases highlight the subjective experience of the disorder far more robustly than the euphoria of mania, despite its consequences. Interestingly, the degree of insight in people with psychotic and non-psychotic bipolar disorder has been found to be unrelated to age, gender, educational level, or history of hospitalization (Yen et al., 2002).

Insight is a complex concept, with numerous definitions having been offered as to what it comprises and how it should be measured. However, insight is generally recognized as multi-faceted, and in bipolar disorder includes awareness of having a mental health problem, awareness of particular symptoms (e.g. anhedonia, asociality, or pressured speech), acknowledgement of symptoms as part of the disorder and not due to other causes (e.g. "normal" adolescence or substance use), appropriate emotional or behavioral responses to symptoms, and awareness of the need for treatment (Sackeim, 1998; Pini et al., 2001; Mintz et al., 2003). It is important to note that these different dimensions of insight can vary for the person during the course of the disorder, and that people may have partial insight involving degrees of awareness of the various components.

Insight in first-episode bipolar disorder

Attaining insight may be particularly challenging in first-episode bipolar disorder. While young people may be willing to openly describe their symptoms, they often attribute these to external sources such as stress or substance use, and may be less likely to accept having a mental health problem than people who have experienced multiple episodes. Young people with bipolar disorder may also be more resistant to acknowledging a psychiatric diagnosis than people with other psychiatric diagnoses, as symptoms of a mood disorder may be less obviously "abnormal" than symptoms in some other disorders, such as hearing voices in psychosis.

Challenges to insight in the early phase of bipolar disorder

There are a number of reasons why people in the early phases of bipolar disorder may have poor insight. These include:

- Manic symptoms such as improved mood, energy, and confidence can be enjoyable. Consequently, the experience of mania and hypomania can seem counter-intuitive to the concept of disorders or illnesses involving pain or distress.
- According to cognitive dissonance theory (Festinger, 1957) and the concept of the manic defense (see Chapter 1), people may guard against beliefs that potentially challenge their sense of independence and competence. Clearly, mental health problems continue to be associated with significant negative stigma. Stigma issues are particularly challenging for young people, in whom the sense of self is still developing and self-esteem may be more dependent on peer opinion. Therefore, refusing to accept a psychiatric diagnosis that identifies a young person not only as different, but potentially defective or vulnerable, appears completely understandable, and may be quite adaptive and even age-appropriate.
- Post-traumatic stress resulting from involuntary hospitalization, depot medication, police involvement, or symptoms themselves, may be particularly distressing and pose a direct threat to the sense of invulnerability that is common in many young people. Again, this may make denial or lack of insight – particularly regarding the likelihood of recurrence – somewhat protective.
- Insight can be seen as at least partly dependent on a person's awareness of how he/she thought, acted, or felt when manic or depressed. Bentall (2003) suggested that poor recall of events and behavior amongst some people recovering from bipolar disorder may be partially determined by the impact of state-dependent memory. Specifically, autobiographical memory is affected by current mood in depressive disorders, and therefore people's recall of manic episodes is often poor. Cassidy et al. (2001) noted that when depressed, people have a tendency to see their weaknesses "with painful clarity," whereas people when manic may have "gross failure in self evaluation" (p. 399). Both of these extremes may be problematic in terms of developing insight.
- Miklowitz (2002) suggested that it can often be difficult for people to disentangle which elements of their mood, thinking, or behavior are due to their personality and which are due to the disorder. He summarized: "Bipolar disorder can be difficult to distinguish from the normal ups and downs of human life" (p. 55). Clearly, denial or minimization of particular symptoms or behaviors is understandable in this context, particularly during adolescence, where mood fluctuation may be common.
- Learning is characteristically experience-based and reinforced by repetition. While recurrent episodes increase an individual's acceptance of the possibility that they may have the disorder, this may be unlikely early in the course of the disorder.

- In some psychiatric disorders, there is an implication that poor insight might be neuropsychologically mediated, and occur outside the person's awareness (McGorry & McConville, 1999). Insight may therefore be related to cognitive deficits experienced by some individuals. It is unclear as to the degree to which poor insight in young people with bipolar disorder with associated psychotic features may be similar to insight in individuals with non-affective psychosis.

Costs and benefits associated with the development of insight

Insight has been viewed for some time as an important goal, if not a prerequisite, in the treatment of people with bipolar disorder. However, a person's understanding of their disorder and their degree of insight can have both positive and negative consequences.

As discussed above, lack of insight can at times be adaptive. Positive consequences that can be associated with lack of insight include preventing the person from developing associated depression, which McGlashan and Carpenter (1976) reported occurs in 25% of people following a psychotic episode. Lack of insight can also prevent suicidal ideation, or excessive acceptance of the sick role, sometimes referred to as "engulfment" (Lally, 1989).

However, lack of insight can also result in negative consequences, including increased likelihood of responding to extremes of emotion in ways that could be harmful to the young person or others. Lack of insight is also likely to present a barrier to seeking treatment, as the young person is unlikely to acknowledge any need for intervention.

Good insight has been correlated with a range of positive factors, including better symptomatic recovery and psychosocial outcome in both psychotic disorders (Williams & Collins, 2002; Yen et al., 2002) and mood disorders (Amador et al., 1994; Yen et al., 2005). A study by Ghaemi et al. (2000b) found that while poor initial insight did not correlate with poor recovery in people with bipolar I disorder, lack of improvement in insight over time did correlate with less favorable outcomes.

Lack of illness awareness and insight has also been found to be positively correlated with medication adherence in bipolar disorder (Scott & Pope, 2002; Yen et al., 2005). However, it has been suggested that for psychotic disorders, insight alone is "neither necessary nor sufficient" to ensure medication adherence (McGorry & McConville, 1999, p. 136). This appears similar for bipolar disorder, as some young people appear to have little insight but continue to take medication, whereas others refuse to take medication despite having good insight.

Adaptation, identity, and sense of self

Bipolar disorder can involve a significant challenge to one's sense of self, particularly for young people. By definition, the disorder involves fluctuations between extremes of mood, thought, behavior, and levels of confidence, which can make it hard for a young person to feel a coherent sense of self. Onset of the disorder during late adolescence or early adulthood can be particularly difficult given that this is a developmental stage where people are integrating the role of themselves as adults (see "Developmental aspects of bipolar disorder in young people" in Chapter 1). In addition, there is a risk that the person may become fearful of extreme moods whether positive or negative, and avoid particular environments or restrict their affect in situations where this could occur (Kahn, 1990).

As Henry et al. (2002) noted regarding first-episode psychosis, "it is important to be mindful that the person is attempting to compensate, not only for the cognitive and emotional disruptions wrought as result of the trauma of psychotic symptoms, but the assault on self-esteem and identity and the disruption to lifestyle. The person is grappling with the meaning and significance of his or her predicament while still in a highly compromised state" (p. 31). This appears equally relevant to a young bipolar population.

Research has suggested that people can react to being given a diagnosis of bipolar disorder in a number of ways. Common reactions can include rejection of the diagnosis, denial of having the disorder at all (referred to as "sealing over"), attributing symptoms to external sources such as drug use or medication side-effects, or minimizing the impact of the disorder. Others may react by merging the disorder into their lives (referred to as "integration"), having curiosity about symptoms, or wholeheartedly accepting the medical model (Lam et al., 1999; Miklowitz, 2002). A number of people describe anxiety and distress resulting from the challenges the disorder poses to their self-image (Scott, 2001). For some people, "engulfment" – or overacceptance and overidentification with the diagnosis – can occur and result in the person adopting a sick role and disengaging from any challenges or avoiding social contact, work, study or other pursuits that they feel may precipitate a relapse. Ramirez-Basco and Rush (2007) observed that, when given a diagnosis of bipolar disorder, some people also transition through stages of denial, anger, bargaining, depression, and acceptance similar to those described by Kubler-Ross (1970) for experiences of grief.

It is also important for the clinician to consider how a person's sense of self may be impacted by relapse. For example, while the first episode can be dismissed or minimized by a young person, a second episode can be considerably more challenging and harder to ignore, to some indicating that they now "are bipolar" or "have" bipolar disorder. One young woman who attended our service stated after experiencing a second episode: "Bipolar disorder used to be something that 'was.' Now it's something that 'is'."

In our experience, it is not uncommon for young people with bipolar disorder to report difficulties in knowing who they are. In her autobiography, *An Unquiet Mind: A Memoir of Moods and Madness*, Jamison (1995) stated of her own experience with bipolar disorder: "Which of the me's is me? The wild, impulsive, chaotic, energetic, and crazy one? Or the shy, withdrawn, desperate, suicidal, doomed, and tired one? Probably a bit of both, hopefully much that is neither" (p. 68). This confusion about identity is often shared by family and friends, who may at times find it challenging that the young person may present with inconsistent mood, behavior, interests, and energy levels, making a stable relationship difficult at times. This is particularly common for individuals with severe symptoms and few periods of euthymic reference.

Stigma, guilt, and shame

People's beliefs about their mental health problems – particularly self-blame, or feeling "trapped" by the disorder – have been found to impact significantly on levels of hopelessness and likelihood of relapse in psychotic disorders (Gumley et al., 2006; White et al., 2007). Issues around stigma, guilt, and shame also appear prominent in the bipolar population, with this including self-stigma, where individuals internalize and apply prevailing negative attitudes regarding the disorder to themselves. In a study of 206 people recruited through the Manic Depressive Fellowship, Hayward et al. (2002) found that participants appeared strongly aware of stigma and negative social attitudes towards people with mental health problems. Interestingly, while the survey indicated that beliefs about stigma did not appear related to mood state, beliefs about stigma *were* correlated with self-esteem in a bidirectional manner. In other words, low self-esteem could lead to increased concern about stigma and vice versa. Similar issues were identified in another large survey

(Morselli & Elgie, 2003), which found that 54.6% of people with bipolar disorder reported feeling stigmatized.

Stigma is particularly important as it has been found to impact on social and leisure functioning in people with bipolar disorder. For example, research by Perlick et al. (2001) found that bipolar participants who had the greatest concerns about stigma also had the greatest social impairment, even when symptom severity, baseline social adaptation, and sociodemographic factors were controlled for. They concluded: "Patients exercise avoidant coping strategies selectively in anticipation of rejection" (p. 1631).

While stigma can be experienced by any person adapting to a psychiatric diagnosis, it can be particularly prominent in bipolar disorder. Clearly, the aftermath of a manic episode may include having to manage the consequences of impulsive or risk-taking behavior, including damage done to relationships, inappropriate sexual activity, embarrassing behavior, or financial recklessness. Jamison (1995) noted of her own spending sprees when manic: "So, after mania, when most depressed, you're given excellent reason to be even more so" (p. 75). Similarly, depressive symptoms can also result in guilt and shame, with symptoms such as anergia, irritability, or withdrawal often being viewed by the young person him/herself, in addition to others, as laziness or selfishness, and possibly resulting in distress or financial hardship for partners or family members.

As Gilbert (2000) noted, guilt and shame are emotions that can impede a person's ability to seek help, and can instead lead people to withdraw, perpetuating further guilt and shame as well as criticism from others. For example, either self-criticism or criticism from others can result in the person labeling themselves as inferior, expecting criticism, behaving submissively, withdrawing, and then putting themselves at risk of further criticism.

Enhancing insight and psychological adaptation

When working with insight and adaptation, it is important that the clinician is patient and recognizes that much of the difficulty in adjusting to bipolar disorder is understandable when expecting a person to accept a new role which may be devalued and stigmatized. McGorry (1995) suggested that for young people with psychosis, "the task of reaching an equilibrium between adjustment to relapsing illness and maintenance of a secure identity and self esteem usually takes several episodes and often many years" (p. 321). This is equally applicable for young people with bipolar disorder.

McGorry and McConville (1999) suggested: "Denial of illness should be respected during the early stages of recovery and should be challenged carefully, even tangentially and only to the extent that it significantly undermines the aims of safety and relief of acute psychotic symptomatology" (p. 139). Because insight can lead to engulfment for some individuals, Williams and Collins (2002) suggested that psychosocial interventions promoting insight should focus on preventing internalized stigma but should also aim to "promote the development of an identity that can incorporate health-seeking behaviors without destructive role constriction" (p. 98).

Strategies to help young people acquire insight, adapt, and develop a secure sense of self in the wake of the onset of bipolar disorder are presented after the following section, which focuses on assessment of insight and adaptation.

Assessing insight, adaptation, and psychoeducational needs

Henry et al. (2002) described a number of useful assessment questions for clinicians working with young people with psychosis in their manual, Cognitively Oriented Psychotherapy for First-Episode Psychosis (COPE): A Practitioner's Manual. Some of these questions, adapted for bipolar disorder, are presented below. We find such questions valuable in facilitating discussion about a young person's explanatory model, perceived control, insight, and understanding of mental health problems. They can also clarify the impact of the disorder, how the person plans to manage it, and issues around trauma and avoidance. This can affect the choice of intervention strategies that could assist the person's adaptation and their psychoeducational needs. Relevant questions may be used at different times and stages of recovery, as appropriate, and language should be tailored to incorporate the terms the young person uses to refer to their experiences.

- What is the person's theory as to what is happening to them?
- What is the meaning of the disorder for the person?
- Why did he/she think it happened?
- Does he/she have any control over it?
- What knowledge does the person have about mania/depression/bipolar disorder?
- How does the person view him/herself now?
- How does the person think family or friends would describe his/her personality, and has this changed?
- Does the person think he/she is different from how he/she was before developing bipolar disorder?
- What perception does the person have now of his/her future? Has it changed?
- How does the person cope with the impact of hospitalization, the manic or depressive episode, or relapse?
- Is there anything the person avoids because it reminds him/her of being unwell?
- How does the person plan to stay well?

Reproduced and modified with kind permission of Lisa Henry

Psychoeducation

The correlation between truth and happiness is not invariably positive.

Sackeim (1998, p. 11)

In a large survey by the US National Depressive and Manic Depressive Association, one-third of respondents reported that they had waited 10 years or more for an accurate diagnosis (Lish et al., 1994). In Australia, the average lag from symptom onset (age 17.5 years) to diagnosis was 12.5 years (Berk et al., 2007). As a result of this delay in accurate diagnosis, lack of information about etiology and treatment is common for people with bipolar disorder, particularly early in its course.

While there is general acceptance regarding the importance of providing patients with information about their disorder and its treatment, there appears to be a lack of consensus at to what this should comprise and how it should be undertaken. As a result, "psycho-education" is a term that has been used quite broadly to describe a number of different interventions (Tacchi & Scott, 2005).

The major misconception regarding psychoeducation is that providing information to people with mental health difficulties in itself results in positive outcomes, particularly in terms of improved medication adherence. Unfortunately, this is not well supported in the research (Tacchi & Scott, 2005), and the Cochrane database review of psychoeducation in schizophrenia (Pekkala & Merinder, 2008) found improved medication adherence in only one of the ten studies reviewed. Tacchi and Scott (2005) noted that as a bare minimum, information had to be targeted at specific individual needs or concerns, and accompanied by the use of modeling or homework and the use of simple cognitive and behavioral interventions, to produce any sustained benefit.

Some emerging research in bipolar disorder has shown that extensive structured psychoeducation programmes can impact positively on outcome, although there are few well-controlled studies. Colom et al. (2003) described a randomized controlled trial of group psychoeducation versus treatment as usual for people with bipolar disorder. It is notable that their intervention comprised 21 sessions lasting 90 minutes each, and involved significantly more than simply providing information, instead covering 4 main areas: awareness of the disorder, treatment adherence, early detection of prodromal symptoms, and encouraging lifestyle regularity. Colom et al. found that their intervention helped prevent episodes of elation, mixed episodes, and depression, and reduced the number of hospitalizations and the number of days the person spent in hospital. Similarly, a recent review by Gonzalez-Pinto et al. (2004) found evidence suggesting that psychoeducation may reduce the number of manic relapses, increase knowledge of bipolar disorder and lithium, improve attitudes towards treatment, and lead to increased medication adherence. Again, however, a fairly broad definition of psychoeducation appears to have been used, with some of the effective studies reported having utilized cognitive techniques, recognition of early signs of relapse, and behavioral interventions to enhance medication adherence.

It appears, therefore, that successful psychoeducation requires interventions designed to create behavioral change, which may also include encouraging self-discovery and helping people find information themselves. It is also likely that the process by which positive outcomes occur is more complex than simply didactically providing young people with information about bipolar disorder.

Content and mode of psychoeducation

Current psychoeducation approaches often include providing written material, videos, or DVDs, or recommending websites regarding bipolar disorder. A recent study indicated that around 84% of people with bipolar disorder were keen to be given such materials (Lewis, 2005). It is also notable that 88% of people with bipolar disorder in a large survey rated receiving information about the disorder "extremely useful or reasonably useful" (Morselli & Elgie, 2003).

Before commencing psychoeducation, thorough assessment of the young person's understanding of their disorder is essential. Specifically, it is important for clinicians to gauge insight, develop an understanding of the young person's explanatory model, and be aware of any potential threat that psychoeducation may pose to self-esteem. This provides a platform for psychoeducation to be delivered in a sensitive manner.

The type of psychoeducation undertaken should reflect the person's stage of disorder, as the messages provided at onset may need to differ to those conveyed later in the course of the disorder. Psychoeducation also needs to be tailored to what the person is ready to hear, and needs to be part of a process of engagement (see Chapter 2).

A handout for use with young people with bipolar disorder is available in Appendix 1, and a handout for families is provided in Appendix 2. However, when providing any written information to young people and their families, it is important to guide them through it. Care should be taken to personalize the information and to obtain feedback about how the client or their family believe specific information may or may not apply to them. In addition, after this face-to-face process, the individual (and family if appropriate) is encouraged to re-read it and to bring questions back to further meetings to clarify any issues or to talk more about specific concerns relating to the content (Scott, 2001).

The internet has also become a place for people to seek information and help, and its use and acceptability as a medium for information on a range of physical and mental health issues is well documented (Fox et al., 2000). A Harris poll of 2000 adults in the United States found that depression, anxiety, and bipolar disorder accounted for 42% of health issues searched on the web (Taylor, 1999). Therefore, it is often useful to inquire as to what young people have seen online and how they view this information. Because the quality of information available on the internet is variable, discussion can also provide an opportunity to correct any misinformation.

Content of psychoeducation in the early phase of bipolar disorder

While clinicians should consider the likely impact of the information they provide to a young person with bipolar disorder and tailor psychoeducation to the individual's needs and stage of recovery, psychoeducation can include discussion of:

- Information about bipolar disorder and diagnosis.
- Information about symptoms of mania, hypomania, depression, and mixed episodes.
- Prevalence of various mental health problems, particularly highlighting the prevalence of depression and mood disorders in young people.
- The etiology of bipolar disorder (acknowledging genetic, biological, and psychosocial factors).
- The role of various clinicians in the treating team (e.g. case manager, therapist, or doctor).
- The role of medication (including its prophylactic function), and medication side-effects.
- The role of psychosocial treatments.
- The importance of structure, balance in daily activities, and sleep.
- How to manage the disorder on a day-to-day basis.
- What to expect during recovery.
- The role of the young person him/herself and the family in the recovery process.
- Ways to prevent relapse.
- Expectations and fears regarding the future.
- Examples of prominent people who have bipolar disorder or unipolar depression and lead successful lives. This can enhance optimism.

Typically, psychoeducation interventions for people with bipolar disorder have utilized a vulnerability-stress model (Zubin & Spring, 1977), which can integrate a number of biological, psychological, and social factors in the etiology and treatment of the disorder. The flexibility of this model generally allows the young person's own explanatory model of their experience to be incorporated relatively easily. Such an approach can foster a collaborative working relationship where people do not feel blamed for developing the disorder and are seen as having a significant role in their own recovery.

In practical terms, the stress-vulnerability model can be illustrated through using metaphors such as a bridge or an overflowing bucket (Brabban & Turkington, 2002). In the bridge metaphor, the onset of mental or physical health difficulties such as diabetes, anxiety, depression, or bipolar disorder occurs when the stress (i.e. "weight" or "traffic") placed on the person (i.e. the "bridge") exceeds its structural strength. Further discussion can focus on what influences the strength of the bridge (e.g. the person's resources, social support, attributional style, and family history) and what constitutes the weight placed on it (e.g. stress, illicit substance use, alcohol, significant life events, and unstable social rhythms).

In the overflowing bucket metaphor, a first episode or relapse of mood symptoms can be described in terms of the person's "bucket becoming too full." This can be represented visually by drawing a bucket and showing increased levels of water through a combination of contributory factors, each of which adds a different volume depending on the individual. This process is done collaboratively with the young person being asked to identify factors they believe may have contributed to the development of their symptoms, and to estimate how much each of these may have contributed. For example, some people may have a significant part of their bucket already full through a strong family history of mental health disorders, with only minimal substance use or stress resulting in the onset of symptoms. In comparison, other people may have little family history but have used a significant amount of illicit substances or have experienced excessive or multiple life stressors, combined with sleep deprivation and a perfectionistic cognitive style.

Importantly, when using the bucket metaphor to describe the stress-vulnerability model, it can be shown that the water level can be reduced by drilling a hole in the bucket, or that the size of the bucket can be increased. It can be explained that this can occur through medication adherence, and by utilizing biopsychosocial interventions such as understanding the disorder, stress management, work on unhelpful schemas, social rhythm regulation, and avoiding illicit substances or alcohol. Similarly, if using the bridge metaphor, therapeutic work can be seen to focus both on reducing the traffic on the bridge and increasing its structural integrity.

Case studies 3.1 and 3.2: the bucket metaphor

Ethan stated that prior to his first manic episode, his parents had separated and he had begun smoking cannabis. He also reported having a premorbid cognitive style that was highly self-critical, and that he tended to become preoccupied with perceived failures. In this way he was able to identify possible environmental, biological, and psychological factors contributing to his episode, as represented in Figure 3.1.

Figure 3.2 shows a bucket representing factors that another young person with bipolar disorder, Emily, identified as possible contributors to her first manic episode. Emily described how her symptoms had occurred in the context of a strong family history, with her mother and sister having been diagnosed with bipolar disorder, and a maternal and paternal grandparent having experienced unipolar depression. Emily also noted that she tended to have extremely high expectations of herself and was facing exams, for which she had been studying late into the night in the weeks prior to becoming manic.

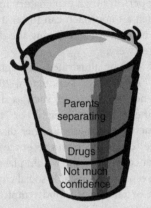

Figure 3.1 Biopsychosocial buckets – Ethan.

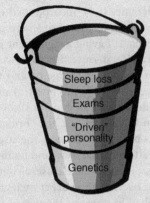

Figure 3.2 Biopsychosocial buckets – Emily.

Case study 3.3: discussing diagnosis and introducing the bucket metaphor – James

James was a 21-year-old man who had an uncle with a diagnosis of bipolar disorder. James presented with a 2-week acute manic episode requiring inpatient admission. His manic episode occurred in the context of several months of dysthymic mood and some brief episodes of undiagnosed depression. He was well engaged with his therapist and the following discussion occurred during their fifth session together.

THERAPIST: "What do you feel like putting on the agenda for today James?"

JAMES: "I wanted to ask why all that stuff happened to me and why I ended up in hospital. And I also want to know what my diagnosis is."

THERAPIST: "James, I'm really keen to discuss these things with you, but I wonder if I can ask first what you think has been going on?" (*The therapist uses an open question and non-medicalized language to facilitate discussion around James' explanatory model before offering his own.*)

JAMES: "I'm not sure, but my mum thinks it might be bipolar disorder."

THERAPIST: "What do you think?"

JAMES: "I'm not sure."

THERAPIST: "What do you think people mean when they talk about 'bipolar disorder'?"

JAMES: "I'm not sure, but I think it's got something to do with feeling really energetic."

THERAPIST: "For some people, I think that's exactly what it's like. Can I ask though, you told me that you have an uncle who has been diagnosed with bipolar disorder. Do you know anyone else who has bipolar disorder, or have you heard much about bipolar disorder?" (*Assessing James' knowledge of the disorder and any associated stereotypes.*)

JAMES: "No. Not really."

THERAPIST: "What has it been like for your uncle?" (*Assessing potential concerns, particularly if James' uncle has had a negative experience with symptoms or treatment.*)

JAMES: "I think pretty bad at the start. He was picked up by the police and was out wandering in the streets. He also seemed really sad a lot of the time before it all happened. My mum said no-one knew what was going on for ages . . . But he's going well now."

THERAPIST: "Have there been things that have happened with you that have been similar to what happened with your uncle?"

JAMES: "Yeah, I've obviously been pretty speedy too and I was feeling really shit for a while before that. But I didn't get in any trouble with the police."

THERAPIST: "So there are some similarities, but your experiences have also been different?" (*Emphasizing that not all people with the diagnosis are the same.*)

JAMES: "Yeah."

THERAPIST: "I wonder if we could have a look at a list of some of the symptoms of bipolar disorder to help us figure out if that might be what has been going on. Does that sound OK?"

JAMES: "Yeah." (*Therapist and James look at the manic symptoms described in Appendix 1.*)

THERAPIST: "Were any of these things happening with you, when you were in hospital?"

JAMES: "Eh . . . (*looking at list*) I was definitely full of energy, and it was hard to concentrate on stuff. A few people said I was talking very fast and I got annoyed pretty easily too. I was also doing some stupid stuff like getting that tattoo and buying all that stuff. Yeah, I think I probably had most of these things."

THERAPIST: "Some people would call that a manic episode. Some people also have times when their mood feels quite low. Can we go through a different list and see if you've had any of these things?" (*Therapist goes to depressive symptoms list in Appendix 1.*)

JAMES (*looking at depressive symptoms list*): "Yeah, I think I had quite a few of these too. I felt pretty sad and slowed down for a few months before I went all speedy."

THERAPIST: "So it looks like you have had some manic symptoms and maybe some symptoms of depression, so bipolar disorder is one possible diagnosis. We try not to focus too much on diagnosis this early in a person's contact with us, as it's often really hard to tell what's going on, and a lot of people's diagnoses change over time. The important thing is that it doesn't change how we work together. The medicine you are taking will be the same, and we will still work on helping you with some of the difficult things that have been happening. James, going back to your other question, why do you think these things have happened to you?"

JAMES: "I'm not sure. I was using a lot of drugs back then and I was pretty stressed at college. Could it maybe also have anything to do with my uncle having it?"

THERAPIST: "Drugs, stress, and family factors could all have played a part . . . Was there anything else going on for you at the time?" (*This allows for elaboration around explanatory models.*)

JAMES: "I wasn't sleeping much and I felt like I was racing about all the time, like my uncle used to do."

THERAPIST: "OK. I'm thinking we can try to put all this together. Sometimes people talk about 'genetic vulnerability,' which means that it might be more likely for someone to get the kind of symptoms you had if other family members have had them. Have you heard of that before?"

JAMES: "Yeah."

THERAPIST: "I also remember you telling me before that you have always tended to push yourself really hard to do well, at school and sport, and that you tend to get down on yourself if you feel you've done badly. Does that sound right?"

JAMES (*smiling*): "Definitely."

THERAPIST: "I wonder if that might be important, because you had exams coming up and had only been sleeping about three hours per night for the three or four days before we first saw you. Taking drugs probably also had an impact and it might be that a combination of these factors all contributed to you getting 'speedy.' What do you think? Does that seem possible?" (*Normalizing the experience and also suggesting an explanatory model that may reduce the perceived unpredictability of the episode.*)

JAMES: "Yeah. I suppose there was a lot going on."

THERAPIST: "Sometimes we use an example of a bucket to describe how it is usually a combination of things that lead to people being 'full of energy' and 'speedy.' (*Utilizing James' expressions. Therapist draws 'empty bucket' [see Appendix 3] on whiteboard.*) So for some people, there might be a really strong family vulnerability and when you add stress, plus no sleep, the water floods over the top. Does that make any sense?"

JAMES: "Yeah. It does."

THERAPIST: "James, can we list the things you think filled up your bucket?"

JAMES: "Probably all the things we talked about . . . I was using drugs, I was worried about how things were going at college and my exams, my uncle had all this stuff, and I wasn't sleeping much too." (*The therapist adds the etiological factors identified by James to the bucket on the whiteboard, showing it overflowing.*)

THERAPIST: "The good thing though is that in the same way that the bucket can become full and overflow, we can drain it by drilling a hole in the bottom (*indicating on diagram*). We drill the hole by making sure we can work to stop your stress levels from getting too high. We can do that by looking at some thoughts you may have had which might not be helpful and also maybe looking at helping you stay off the drugs you were taking which might have had an unsettling effect on your mood. Part of it can also be helping to make sure that you're sleeping the right amount, eating, and exercising OK, and having the right dose of a medicine that helps you. Am I explaining that OK?"

JAMES: "Yeah."

THERAPIST: "What do you think of all that, James?" (*Gauging James' reaction and offering opportunity for clarification.*)

JAMES: "It all sounds OK. I just wasn't that sure what was going on before, but it kind of makes sense that I got pretty stressed and acted a bit weird because of everything that was going on."

Working to enhance psychological adaptation and reduce stigma, guilt, and shame

There are many clinical strategies that clinicians will already utilize when working on adaptation or guilt and shame. Rather than repeat these techniques here, we focus on an additional method, the repertory grid, which has proved useful for younger adults and also offers the clinician a structured assessment tool.

Assessing adaptation: repertory grids

Repertory grids can be helpful in working with adaptation and stigma in bipolar disorder, and have been described in work with young people experiencing psychotic disorders (Henry et al., 2002) and adults with affective disorders (Boker et al., 2000). In this technique, the young person is asked to select three concepts from a list such as: "yourself now," "yourself before bipolar disorder," "how you would like to be," "your best friend," "yourself in the future," "yourself when manic," "yourself when depressed," or "someone with bipolar disorder." If the young person chooses "current self," "past self," and "manic self," he or she is then asked to describe a way in which the first concept differs from the other two. For example, the young person may respond that their current self differs from their past self, and self when manic, by being "shy" rather than "confident." The young person is then asked to give other examples of how their current self differs from their past and manic selves, which may include "alone" as opposed to "popular," and "boring" rather than "creative." This procedure is repeated for other combinations of three concepts, and results in a list of "contrasts" (rather than just opposites) being generated. The clinician then asks the young person to plot these on a 1–7 point scale, or Likert scale.

While we recognize that this approach may be too complex to use with some young people, a simplified version can be undertaken. Specifically, the young person can be given a pre-written list of some common themes that are relevant in adaptation to bipolar disorder, an example of which is provided in Appendix 4. The young person is asked to complete one of these sheets describing him/herself "before bipolar disorder" and another describing how he/she views him/herself "now."

While there are numerous ways of analyzing repertory grids for research purposes, we use them more as a clinical tool. Specifically, responses can promote fruitful discussion regarding how the young person feels bipolar disorder has affected them and their future, and also clarify preconceived ideas and stigma relating to the disorder. Repertory grids can be repeated at different phases of recovery to track changes over time. It can also be worthwhile to ask the young person to select a friend or family member to complete these grids, as these can yield interesting results. However, time should be taken with the young person and the person completing the form to "debrief" and discuss the content afterwards, particularly if negative changes are noted.

The "Views on manic depression questionnaire" (Hayward et al., 2002) can also provide a framework for raising issues around adaptation and stigma, and a modified version is included as Appendix 5. This measure is designed to assess the person's perceptions of the impact of bipolar disorder on their functioning, particularly in work and relationships, and also their beliefs about societal stigma towards the disorder.

Kahn (1990) noted the importance of acknowledging both symbolic and realistic losses that may have resulted from bipolar disorder, and it can be important to recognize and address this in work with young people. Goodwin and Jamison (1990) quoted a previously hypomanic patient who stated: "When I am my present 'normal' self, I am far removed from when I have been my liveliest, most productive, most intense, most outgoing, and effervescent. In short, for myself, I am a hard act to follow" (p. 730). We commonly hear young people express such beliefs, particularly as some aspects of mania or hypomania such as increased energy, confidence, or creativity are extremely enjoyable. Therefore part of adaptation may involve helping the young person manage to cope with "missing" their previously manic or hypomanic self.

Clearly, discussions around stigma, guilt, and loss can be associated with distress, should only be discussed in the context of a strong therapeutic relationship, and generally occur in the middle to latter stages of therapy. However, it can be useful to utilize cognitive techniques that help the person identify the role that shame may have in maintaining their low mood. Identifying particular situations, interactions, or people that appear to lead to feelings of guilt can also be valuable, either to help the person prepare for them, or avoid them if appropriate. We encourage young people to identify specific cognitions which may be part of their guilt and manage these in a similar way to that of unhelpful depressive cognitions (see Chapter 5). This can include reality-checking as to whether the person would treat one of their friends differently if they were given the diagnosis, and testing the validity of beliefs such as people with bipolar disorder being unable to find a partner or maintain employment or study. Gilbert (2000) advocated that it can be valuable to encourage people to challenge their "inner bully" (p. 152). This consists of the person identifying in what ways they bully themselves, and being encouraged to have a dialogue with their critical self, identify what thinking errors may be present (e.g. "black and white thinking"), and challenge these with believable counter-arguments.

It is encouraging to note that while Morselli and Elgie (2003) found that most of their participants (86.8%) who had been diagnosed with bipolar disorder reported that it had impacted heavily on their life in the past, significantly fewer (48.6%) described that this was an ongoing concern. This would suggest that many people find ways of adapting to, or managing, the disorder.

Post-traumatic growth

While much research has concentrated on distress and loss resulting from diagnosis of a mental health disorder, in recent years a literature is also emerging on the concept of post-traumatic growth. While to date this has generally focused on adaptation following disaster or physical trauma, we suggest this can be applied to psychological trauma, including the experience of first-episode bipolar disorder.

The post-traumatic growth literature has identified that following the initial impact of a traumatic event, between 40% and 70% of people report positive elements resulting from it. This can include changes to how the person views themselves, how relationships are perceived, or how the person sees life (Calhoun & Tedeschi, 1999; Woodward & Joseph, 2003). Following major physical trauma, participants interviewed by Turner and Cox (2004) identified that "determination," "motivation," and setting stepwise goals allowed them to view the world differently, often more positively (p. 6). Participants also reported that they felt they had become more tolerant, patient, and had re-prioritised what was important in their lives. Importantly, control and independence appeared significant for the participants Turner and Cox interviewed, and despite needing the care of others when acutely unwell, "none had any intention of allowing dependency states in their future" (p. 5). Similarly, research by Dunkley et al. (2007) described a 22-year-old man with bipolar disorder, and while clearly describing initial distress associated with his symptoms, he was able to report: "You appreciate life a hell of a lot more and I don't think it is something you can have unless you've been through what I've been through" (p. 9).

Joseph and Linley (2004) suggested that clinicians can facilitate post-traumatic growth through being aware that adversity and trauma can result in growth, while recognizing that trauma does not necessarily lead to growth in all people. This may prevent therapists inadvertently blaming clients who do not react positively to their negative event. Joseph and Linley also advised that clinicians should be careful not to imply that the event in itself is positive, but instead emphasize that it is the person's *adaptation* which is important. They concluded: "It is evident that the concept of meaning is central to understanding adjustment to threatening events" (p. 1045).

Work which focuses on growth can be extremely valuable, even after a first episode. However, it appears important that the clinician is watchful for overoptimism or unrealistic overconfidence from the young person, particularly if this occurs too early in the course of therapy. An overly positive style early in recovery, in which the young person fails to acknowledge the impact of the disorder, may be indicative of pseudo-recovery or "sealing over." However, over time, a number of young people genuinely appear to manage their disorder extremely well, and the experience can result in the person reconsidering their goals and hopes for the future in a positive way. It is not uncommon for some young people to describe wishing to pursue more compassionate or altruistic career or study paths following their experience of bipolar disorder.

Case study 3.4: explanatory models and adaptation – Tony

Tony was a 25-year-old man who had recently developed bipolar disorder. His mother and sister had both been diagnosed with bipolar disorder, and Tony had cared for his mother – which included administering her medication – during the previous eight years, prior to developing symptoms himself. Tony made a reasonably rapid recovery from his acute manic symptoms, but developed depressive symptoms around the time he gained increasing insight that he might also have bipolar disorder.

It was important for the therapist to be aware that Tony was likely to have significant concerns around having the same diagnosis as his mother and sister. It was also important to assess the impact on Tony of his change of role from carer to being cared for by his mother, who was reasonably stable at the time of Tony's acute symptoms. This appeared to contribute significantly to the emergence of his depressive symptoms, as he had previously described himself as highly independent, strong, and a carer for others.

Tony's explanatory model focused on having excessive stress at the time of his episode, and that he had also tried smoking marijuana for the first time during the three weeks prior to becoming unwell. Although he initially minimized his likelihood of relapse, he was later concerned that even if he monitored his stress and avoided cannabis, he may be vulnerable to another episode given his family history. He accepted that medication may have offered a "protective layer" against stress, but had become quite anxious and socially withdrawn in an attempt to limit any activities that could precipitate relapse.

Time was spent with Tony discussing what he thought it would mean if he did have bipolar disorder and how he felt this would impact on his life. Particular emphasis was placed on exploring the differences between the disorder for him and for his mother and sister. For example, it appeared very important to discuss how Tony's sister appeared to have little insight, continued to use illicit drugs, and refused medication. His mother appeared to have had an extremely long period of symptoms before her initial treatment. Discussion also highlighted significant differences between the premorbid personality styles of Tony, his mother, and his sister, how each had managed their disorder, and their experience of differing outcomes. The analogy was used that although three different people could all have brown eyes, this may be where their similarities ended in terms of personality or behavior.

While Tony did not initially agree with his diagnosis of bipolar disorder, he accepted that he had experienced a manic episode, and that medication could be helpful in avoiding a relapse, although there was significant negotiation around dosage. It was felt that this was an acceptable level of agreement, and allowed for a good therapeutic relationship.

Time was also spent looking at how Tony viewed changes to himself. Repertory grid work indicated that he viewed his past self globally in very positive terms, particularly regarding confidence and independence. However, after his manic episode, he experienced significant guilt and shame around his behavior when unwell, particularly promiscuity, which was highly unusual for him. He also reported a negative view of his future self, perhaps largely due to overidentification with, and hypervigilance regarding, his symptoms.

Due to expressing confusion as to who he "was," time was spent in sessions with Tony and his family discussing his previous personality traits. These family meetings were at times emotional, but helpful, and indicated that family members viewed Tony very positively, both currently and prior to developing his manic episode, something they had not been able to express to him before.

Although it took several months, Tony appeared able to integrate having experienced a mood disorder for which he had to make some changes to his life – including monitoring stress levels, taking medication, and avoiding illicit substances – without this impacting significantly on his sense of self. Interestingly, towards the end of therapy, he was able to describe some positive aspects of having experienced a mood disorder including his belief that it had made him a more sensitive and less self-absorbed person, particularly towards his mother, who he had cared for but previously seen as something of a burden. Tony also described that having insight into manic symptoms actually helped his relationships with his mother and sister, and allowed him to be more patient, less frustrated, and more empathic towards them. He also noted that he became better at allowing others to care for him at times, thus creating more of a balance in his relationships.

A strong emphasis on supporting functional recovery is also important to assist adaptation to the disorder and development or maintenance of a positive sense of self. The next section of this chapter discusses ways to promote functional recovery in young people with bipolar disorder.

Functional recovery

Most research indicates that functional outcome is poor following bipolar disorder. While around 90% of young people achieve syndromal recovery at 12 months after their first manic episode, only 39% reach functional recovery (Conus et al., 2006). Klerman et al. (1992) found that over 25% of people with bipolar disorder under the age of 65 were receiving disability payments.

There are a number of factors which could contribute to this poor functional outcome, not least that research indicates that over 40% of young people with bipolar disorder continue to experience subsyndromal depressive or hypomanic symptoms even when apparently in remission (Conus et al., 2006). Morriss (2002) suggested that inter-episode symptoms are frequently missed by clinicians because some standardized measures are not sensitive to low levels of symptomatology. Furthermore, people with bipolar disorder have a tendency to minimize and under-report symptoms unless directly asked about them. Therefore, even when the young person presents well, the clinician should inquire about the existence of any residual symptoms, rather than assume a full recovery. However, this should be managed sensitively in order to avoid hypervigilance.

Social functioning

For many young people, bipolar disorder has an impact on social functioning, and a number report social withdrawal due to ongoing symptoms or concerns about stigma relating to their disorder. A recent study by Pope et al. (2007) found that the 2 best predictors of poor social functioning in people with bipolar disorder were premorbid neuroticism (which accounted for nearly 24% of the variance) and current level of depressive symptomatology (accounting for 9% of the variance). They hypothesized that neuroticism may impact on social functioning because it has been associated with higher levels of attention to negative information about the self, and therefore it could be an important focus for cognitive treatment.

Another factor that can impact on psychosocial recovery, which may often be missed by clinicians, is cognitive impairment. In a recent paper, Martinez-Aran et al. (2007) reported that previous studies have identified comorbid substance use, medication side-effects, psychotic symptoms, low premorbid functioning, a higher number of episodes, and earlier onset of the disorder as factors impacting on functional outcome. However, in their study of 77 euthymic bipolar patients, poor verbal memory was the best predictor of impaired psychosocial functioning. They noted specifically that difficulty remembering names and conversations impacted negatively on both occupational and social functioning. While this study requires replication, it highlights the need for clinicians to assess the cognitive functioning of their bipolar patients. We find anecdotally that a number of young people report these difficulties with memory, making participating in conversations and large social encounters particularly challenging. One young man told us: "I can't keep up with the conversation any more. I feel like I'm just an observer now when I'm with my mates."

Mental health support groups can be helpful in the short term to assist people to reintegrate socially following the acute phase of bipolar disorder, and young people often report it being helpful to know that they are "not alone." However, there are risks that people may remain "stuck" if using these exclusively. In a survey of people who had remained asymptomatic, Russell and Browne (2005) quoted one man with bipolar disorder who was critical of mental health support groups: "You mix with the same people as in hospital. You drink coffee, smoke, and talk about the same things – hospital admission, drug reactions, and Centrelink (Australian unemployment benefits agency). These groups do not encourage you to get on with your life and get back to work" (p. 191).

Russell and Browne (2005) noted that people who self-reported a successful outcome following bipolar disorder described having used a range of social networks including partners, family members, friends, colleagues, religious groups, and mental health services and groups. Therefore, encouragement to maintain contact with a variety of people, including those not involved in the mental health system, in addition to identifying barriers to social activity, appears essential.

Vocational and educational functioning

Due to the age of onset of bipolar disorder, disruption to schooling, tertiary study, or early workplace training is common. While some of the difficulties in returning to work or study after a first episode are described above, a pervasive and at times unhelpful belief among many young people and their families is that a return to social or vocational activity should only occur when the person has made a full recovery. This belief is understandable and may be a by-product of the stress-vulnerability model, as people may deliberately avoid activity for fear of relapse. However, assisting the young person to return to education or work early can be an extremely important treatment goal, not least as unemployment has been associated with increased suicide rates in people with mood disorders (Brown et al., 2000). Vocational or educational involvement can help the young person regain a sense of role and purposeful activity, provide structure for social rhythms, challenge negative self-beliefs which can result from inactivity, increase self-confidence, and prevent self-stigmatization which may result from overidentifying with a psychiatric diagnosis.

Fowler (personal communication, 2007) has emphasized the importance of practical assistance and support to facilitate a return to employment for young people with mental health issues, rather than focusing solely on office-based psychological therapy. While therapy may involve finding ways to manage anxiety and loss of self-confidence, a practical focus should be maintained, as excessive time spent in discussion can reinforce secondary morbidity and loss of self-efficacy, and make returning to work or study more daunting. Practical support can involve liaison with employment, educational, and voluntary services to assist people in returning to premorbid functioning as soon as is reasonable without risking relapse. Ongoing contact with employers or schools, and if helpful, actually attending appointments with the young person, can be also very valuable, as can providing information about bipolar disorder to these agencies if the young person is agreeable to this.

In addition to impaired self-esteem, concerns about how to explain absence from work or study can be difficult, and unfortunately the longer the young person takes to return to work or study, the more this worry can be reinforced. Therefore, possible explanations regarding the absence should be considered with the young person, in addition to the level of disclosure that they would be comfortable with, and with whom they will discuss what they have experienced. This may result in the young person utilizing explanations such as "I was sick," "I got pretty stressed," "I had a health problem," "I had women's problems," "the doctor said I should take some time off," or "it's kind of personal, but I'm OK now," to explain their absence. It can be valuable for the therapist to role-play a coercive friend/colleague/boss/student/teacher in order to prepare the young person for more intrusive questioning. This will allow the young person to be confident that they will only disclose what they are willing to.

Supporting return to work

Wallace et al. (1999) and Wallace and Tauber (2004) described a detailed, structured approach to help people with mental health problems maintain employment. This included:
- Examining the costs and benefits of working.
- Identifying specific aspects of what the job would involve.
- Identifying potential stressors.
- Learning how to use general problem-solving.
- Managing mental and physical health (including substance use).
- Maintaining positive contact with supervisors and colleagues.
- Managing social situations with colleagues.
- Identifying what supports can be accessed both at work and outside of work.

Addressing some of these issues in one-to-one therapy sessions, and role-playing specific work or study situations, can be valuable. It also appears essential to ensure that these skills generalize to the real world by encouraging in vivo work, and asking the young person to practice in real world settings.

A further component of intervention to assist young people to return to work or study is ensuring positive sleep patterns. We find that a number of young people who have been unemployed for a length of time develop a reversed sleep cycle. This can make it particularly challenging to attend work or study that commences early in the morning. Problems with sleep often result in the person being late or unable to attend their first few days, which can put their job, or position on a course, in jeopardy. While it can sometimes be possible to help the young person negotiate flexible work hours, as part of planning for return to work or study we encourage people to begin readjusting their sleep patterns in the weeks prior to their first day, taking a graded approach. For example, if a person typically wakes at midday, we may ask them to set their alarm for 11.30 am the following day, 11 am the day after, 10.30 am the day after that, and so on until they reach the time they need to rise. In order to encourage this, we typically ask the young person to schedule something pleasurable to do first thing, to offer an incentive to get up. This has included activities such as watching a favorite episode of a DVD, having a favorite CD ready to play, or playing an enjoyable videogame. It may be necessary for the clinician to call the young person at the arranged time over the first few days, to ensure they have woken, but if possible, we encourage the young person to make a very brief telephone call to their clinician to inform them that they have woken up.

Conclusions

- Insight is often poor in bipolar disorder, with many young people initially having a limited understanding of the condition and its treatment.
- Poor insight has been correlated with poorer medication adherence and less favorable outcomes in bipolar disorder. However, insight is a complex concept, may have a strong protective role for the individual, and should be managed sensitively.
- There are a number of psychoeducational handouts, videotapes, DVDs, and websites that describe biological, psychological, and social aspects of etiology and treatment of bipolar disorder. However, such materials should only be provided after significant discussion has occurred, and the clinician has a clear understanding of the person's explanatory model, their stage of recovery, and the likely impact of providing such information.
- Effective psychoeducation goes beyond simple didactic provision of information about bipolar disorder, and should instead encompass behavioral change and encouragement of self-discovery about the disorder.
- Clinicians should be aware that guilt, loss, and stigma can be significant factors accompanying bipolar disorder, and should sensitively screen for and address these if present.
- It appears essential that social, vocational, and educational functioning is encouraged, and that return to work or study is framed as an important goal of recovery. The clinician should focus on assessing and managing inter-episode mood symptoms, cognitive difficulties, anxiety, and sleep difficulties, all of which may impact on the young person's ability to return to their previous level of functioning.

Medication adherence

The major clinical problem in treating manic-depressive illness is not that there are not effective medications – there are – but that patients so often refuse to take them.

Jamison, *An Unquiet Mind: A Memoir of Moods and Madness* (1995, p. 6)

Medication adherence can be a vital component in the treatment of bipolar disorder, as people who are fully adherent are more likely to achieve syndromal recovery than those who are non-adherent or partially adherent (Keck et al., 1998). In addition, adherence with mood stabilizers such as lithium has been found to significantly reduce the likelihood of attempted or completed suicide in people with mood disorders (Muller-Oerlinghausen et al., 1996; Sachs, 2003; Colom et al., 2005).

Conversely, non-adherence with prescribed medication has been found to influence risk of relapse. For example, a review by Colom et al. (2005) noted that rapid discontinuation of lithium was associated with relapse rates of 50% in the 3 months following cessation, compared with less than 10% in people who continued taking prophylactic medication. Furthermore, Strakowski et al. (1998) noted that 60–80% of people admitted to hospital due to a manic episode had been non-adherent in the previous month.

Unfortunately, poor medication adherence is a longstanding problem in bipolar disorder, and continues to represent a significant challenge. In John Cade's (1949) landmark paper, the first case study he reported was a man whose manic symptoms improved significantly with lithium, following which the man returned to work, ceased medication, and relapsed within 6 weeks. Reviews by Lingam and Scott (2002), Colom et al. (2005), and Scott and Tacchi (2002) suggested that little has changed, with a consensus that between 40% and 60% of people with bipolar disorder are non-adherent with mood-stabilizing medication (Goodwin & Jamison, 1990; Ramirez-Basco & Rush, 1996; Morselli & Elgie, 2003).

Despite lithium being considered by many clinicians to be required for the course of the person's life, a study of over 1000 people with bipolar disorder found that the mean length of adherence for this medication was only 76 days (Johnson & McFarland, 1996). Rates are similarly low in adolescents and children with bipolar disorder, with recent papers indicating adherence rates for mood stabilizers of between 34% and 66% (Coletti et al., 2005; Drotar et al., 2007).

Medication adherence remains an important treatment goal in early work with young people, particularly as the first episode could provide the best opportunity for effective biological treatment, with evidence that medication effectiveness may be reduced with successive episodes (Gelenberg et al., 1989; Swann et al., 1999). There is also evidence that the subtle but progressive brain changes seen with neuroimaging may be preventable with appropriate early biological treatment (Strakowski et al., 2002).

Reasons for poor medication adherence in bipolar disorder

The reasons why a young person takes, or does not take, mood-stabilizing medication may be partially explained through the "health belief model" (Babiker, 1986) and the "cognitive representation of illness" model (Scott & Tacchi, 2002). These assert that medication adherence is determined by the person's perception of the seriousness of the disorder, his/her perceived susceptibility to it, and what he/she believes may be an effective way to manage it (which may or may not include the use of medication). Clearly, manic or hypomanic symptoms may not result in a person feeling subjectively unwell, could even be enjoyable, and may not be considered a serious health problem by the person experiencing them. Equally, when experiencing a major depressive episode, hopelessness may result in the young person having little optimism about the potential effectiveness of medication.

While the difficulty of achieving good medication adherence has been noted in the adult bipolar population, this can be even more challenging in young people early in the course of the disorder, due to an increased likelihood of "lack of illness awareness." This awareness generally increases with the experience of multiple episodes, particularly relapse following discontinuation of medication, as the individual increasingly acknowledges or can no longer rationalize the presence of these periods of ill health. Following the first episode, young people often minimize symptoms, particularly if acute symptoms resolved quickly, or if they could be attributed to another factor, such as stress or substance use. Young people also understandably underestimate their susceptibility to future episodes (Scott & Tacchi, 2002).

It is also notable that some of the most common factors associated with non-adherence – namely younger age, male gender, experience of fewer episodes, and a prior history of non-adherence (Berk et al., 2004; Drotar et al., 2007) – are common characteristics of a first-episode population. However, most of these factors are not amenable to modification through therapy interventions, and it is increasingly recognized that these do not help clinicians identify specific individuals who may be at risk of non-adherence. Exploring attitudes and expectations regarding medication and treatment is far more likely to identify those at risk of reduced adherence. For example, a survey of over 1000 people with bipolar disorder found that almost half of the respondents indicated that taking medication "bothered" them (Morselli & Elgie, 2003, p. 272). The most commonly reported reasons for stopping medication against medical advice according to this survey were being "tired of taking drugs" (21%), believing "they are useless" (18.9%), and experiencing "disturbing side effects" (18.3%). Scott and Pope (2003) found that the 2 most commonly cited reasons given by people for non-adherence with lithium were not wanting their moods to be controlled by medication, and feeling that medication acted as a regular reminder of having a mental health problem.

Reasons for poor medication adherence in young people with bipolar disorder

- One of the most important reasons for poor medication adherence in bipolar disorder is wishing to avoid the stigma of long-term psychiatric medication, and it being perceived as a daily reminder of having a mental health problem. This is particularly true immediately following the first episode, as many young people may have had little previous contact with any health professionals, with mental health problems being particularly stigmatized.

Due to the importance of peer relationships during adolescence and early adulthood, young people are often concerned about anything that marks them as different from their peer group. As Corsano et al. (2006) concluded from their research involving 330 young people, "psychological well-being, above all during early adolescence, depends on acceptance and integration into the peer group" (p. 350).

- The high prevalence of comorbid disorders, including substance abuse (Swofford et al., 1996), is likely to impact on the probability that a person will be adherent with medication. Tacchi and Scott (2005) identified that comorbid substance and alcohol use were the most important risk factors for non-adherence in people with bipolar disorder. In addition, substance use (particularly amphetamines) at the time of developing a manic episode can allow people to attribute symptoms to intoxication, and lead to rejecting the need for ongoing medication. Attempts at self-medication through substance use may also mean the individual chooses alternative methods to try to contain their symptoms.

- As discussed in Chapter 2 in relation to engagement difficulties, mania and hypomania can be pleasurable, and symptoms may not fit with perceptions of what constitutes an illness or disorder. Therefore medication to manage these may not appear necessary. The predominant polarity therefore impacts on adherence, as individuals presenting with manic episodes are more likely to be non-adherent than those with predominant depression. In a young bipolar population, where anxiety can be prevalent, hypomania and mania can increase self-confidence and enhance beliefs of social competence, with this escape from self-consciousness and self-criticism being a major barrier to engaging with medication.

- A number of young people appear to experience rapid symptomatic improvement within days or weeks of commencing medication. Paradoxically, this can lead to "sealing over" and denial of having the disorder. People often misunderstand the concept of preventive medication use, with "common sense" dictating that medication is only necessary when a person is unwell (e.g. taking painkillers only when experiencing an acute headache).

- Side-effects are common with a number of medications used in the treatment of bipolar disorder. For example, Lam et al. (1999) found that 75% of people taking lithium reported side-effects.

  Some of the least acceptable side-effects, and those most likely to lead to non-adherence, are weight gain and tremor (Goodwin & Jamison, 1990). In the EPPIC young, first-episode bipolar population, weight gain, sedation, slowed motor coordination, and thirst were the main concerns voiced (EPPIC, unpublished data).

  However, Scott and Pope (2002) noted that it was the *fear* of side-effects rather than actual side-effects of mood stabilizers that predicted non-adherence. In another paper, Tacchi and Scott (2005) concluded: "Objective examinations of the prevalence of side effects demonstrate only a weak association between current side effects and adherence" (p. 24). It appears that the specific meaning or importance of the side-effect (e.g. a fear that lithium will impair memory, or that some antipsychotics will lead to weight gain), and the individual's concerns that they will not be able to *manage* the side-effects, are the more common determinants of how an individual copes.

- Medication is not universally effective, and perceived lack of efficacy, particularly in the depressive phase, may lead some people to be non-adherent. Many medications display partial efficacy, resulting in the frequent need for combination strategies. This perceived lack of robust efficacy, and the need to take multiple medications, is likely to impair adherence.

- Manic symptoms including disorganization, impulsivity, and memory difficulties can impact on a person's ability to take medication. Similarly, lack of motivation and hopelessness associated with depression can impact on attendance at appointments, engagement in collaborative work, and the ability to fill prescriptions.

- Rebelling against those who want the person to take medication – particularly parents, doctors, or other authority figures – appears to be a reason for poor medication adherence by some adolescents.

- Lack of insight or denial of the severity of the disorder can be an inherent aspect of mania (Johnson & Leahy, 2004), and is particularly common in the early stages of mania (EPPIC, unpublished data). Greenhouse et al. (2000) found a clear relationship between medication non-adherence and denial of having bipolar disorder. They concluded: "With lower acceptance (and higher denial), adherence scores deteriorated exponentially" (p. 240).

- Some people report fearing losing the sense of creativity that can accompany mania. Jamison (1995) noted: "My manias, at least in their early and mild forms, were absolutely intoxicating states that gave rise to great personal pleasure, an incomparable flow of thoughts and a ceaseless energy" (p. 6).

- Many people experience episodes of depression, dysthymia, or anxiety prior to experiencing mania, and mania may give some relief from these. Therefore, particularly during periods of hypomania, people may be non-adherent due to fear of returning to their depressive state or experiencing symptoms of anxiety. One of the young men with whom we work compared his prevalent dysphoric mood with mania, stating: "It feels like most of the time you're falling to the ground. How often do we get to walk on clouds?" Clearly this is likely to impact on willingness to take medication.

- Negative attitudes towards medication by the young person or important others, including family members, are likely to impact on likelihood of taking medication. Common negative beliefs can include that it is "weak" to take medication or that natural remedies are safer than prescription medications. Fear of becoming "addicted" to, or dependent on, the medication can also contribute to non-adherence. Some people may experience active discouragement from others regarding taking medication, with this occurring especially among parents or friends who have had negative experiences with medication themselves.

- Some cultural or gender issues may impact on likelihood of medication adherence. For example, Australian culture encourages the concept of the "Aussie battler," and the British stereotype of a "stiff upper lip" and "never surrendering" may result in young men in particular often reporting the wish to manage their mood without the assistance of medication.

- We find that many young people initially miss medication doses accidentally rather than intentionally setting out to be non-adherent. Often, forgetting occasional doses of a mood stabilizer is not problematic in the initial few days, and does not lead to immediate relapse, which may perpetuate an individual's belief that they no longer require medication. It may also lead to the young person subjectively experiencing improvement of mood in the short term, due to mild hypomania or reduction of sedation, further reducing their likelihood of remaining adherent.

- Taking medication can, for some young people, act as a daily reminder that they have been unwell, and some may wish to cease taking it to avoid distressing or embarrassing memories, in addition to demonstrating to themselves and others that they no longer have the disorder.

It is important to recognize that there are numerous potential reasons why a young person with bipolar disorder may not adhere to medication. Taking the time to explore an individual's idiosyncratic reasons for non-adherence is crucial and assists in selecting appropriate strategies to attempt to enhance adherence.

Factors which may assist medication adherence in young people with bipolar disorder

Understanding the person's own reasons for non-adherence, and discussing concerns regarding taking medication

This can include discussion around which of the factors described above are present for the young person, or whether other reasons for poor adherence are relevant. Bauer and McBride (2003) described the importance of the individual's cost-benefit analysis in relation to decision-making about whether to accept treatment. Specifically, they suggested that a person's health-related decisions "are always made on the basis of his or her attempt to adapt with the greatest benefit, or least harm to self" (p. 120). They also described the role of the clinician in helping the person understand their decision-making process and assisting in identifying previously unrecognized costs of non-adherence and benefits of adherence.

Scott (2001) suggested this cost-benefit analysis can be operationalized using a four-cell matrix of the advantages and disadvantages of taking and not taking medication (see Appendix 6). This approach allows the clinician to inquire about, and anticipate, individual barriers to adherence.

Recognizing that adherence is not a polarized concept

There is a danger that, particularly when working with young people, clinicians may be at risk of adopting a more authoritarian or directive stance regarding medication adherence, albeit with the intention of helping the young person avoid the distress associated with multiple episodes. Unfortunately, however, with young people, a "doctor knows best" approach is unlikely to be effective, and may simply create further resistance, leading to a cycle in which both the young person and clinician become more entrenched. As Goodwin and Jamison (2007) noted, "it is important not to attempt to control the patient unduly and not to allow medications to become the focus of a power struggle" (p. 872).

To reduce therapist frustration and the likelihood of a conflictual therapeutic relationship, it can be important to recognize that most people experiencing either physical or mental health difficulties are neither fully adherent nor totally non-adherent with medication. Furthermore, adherence can vary within the same person at different times. Colom et al. (2005) have described numerous forms of non-adherence ranging from complete non-adherence (where the person fails to take any prescribed medication), through selective and intermittent non-adherence depending on the type of medication or varying with time, to "abuse" (where the person takes more medication than prescribed). However, partial adherence is the most common form of non-adherence with medication (Cramer & Rosenheck, 1998). It can also be valuable for the clinician to be aware that medication adherence is often no worse in patients with mental health problems than in patients with long-term physical health difficulties (Cramer & Rosenheck, 1998). It is important in work with young people that they have a sense of ownership of the treatment decisions or plan, and motivational interviewing-type techniques are often useful in this regard (see Chapter 8).

It is critically important that the clinician creates an atmosphere in which the young person feels able to discuss their actual levels of adherence freely. Awareness and acceptance that adherence is a flexible concept can be important for the clinician to acknowledge. Similarly, remembering difficulties they may have encountered when trying to change their own behaviors may encourage clinicians to understand that knowing that an activity is likely to improve health does not instantly enable us to sustain a new behavior. Tacchi and Scott (2005) highlight the importance of setting the scene with the client through "normalizing" non-adherence. This can be done by acknowledging that struggling to sustain new behaviors is common (e.g. most people try to lose weight or stop smoking cigarettes several times before finally being able to sustain this change). Following this, it can be important to use non-judgemental questions. For example, inquiring, "do you ever try and cope on your own without your medication?" (in acknowledgement that this is a common reason for choosing not to adhere), rather than bluntly asking, "have you been taking your medication?" is likely to lead to a more helpful and accurate response. Other questions that give a message that "perfect" adherence is not expected may include "how many times have you missed some of your pills in the last week?" or "what has got in the way of you taking medication recently?" These approaches may allow for a dialogue around the person's attitude and behavior towards medication.

Identifying the right medication at the right dose

It is appropriate to try, within the limits of what treatments and medications are known to be effective, to offer a young person some choice between medications as well as agreeing the target of the "minimum effective dose." Regularly re-emphasizing that medication is only one aspect of the intervention being offered is also essential. However, when monitoring the benefits and/or encouraging open dialogue about any difficulties related to medication, clinicians will also want to devise a reliable method of screening for side-effects. Measures such as the UKU side-effect rating scale (Lingjaerde et al., 1987) can be useful, but the clinician should be mindful that extensive checking with side-effect lists may increase rather than reduce the young person's concerns about the use of medication. However, if used appropriately, these can be helpful, provided they are accompanied by clinicians being able to routinely explain methods of coping with identified side-effects that are a nuisance but not dangerous (e.g. sucking sweets or chewing gum to reduce dry mouth), and distinguishing them from those which require active help-seeking (such as marked tremor or even ataxia when lithium levels are at toxic levels). We typically inquire about:

- Light-headedness, dizziness, or fainting.
- Sedation or excessive sleeping.
- Nausea or vomiting.
- Increased appetite or weight gain.
- Stiffness or shaking.
- Muscle pain.
- Skin rashes or acne.
- Dry mouth or thirst.
- Sexual difficulties including erectile dysfunction or menstrual changes.
- Gastrointestinal difficulties including constipation or diarrhoea.

Concerns about weight gain should be addressed early, particularly as the person may initially experience a more sedentary lifestyle following a severe mood episode or hospitalization. Discussion around the importance of maintaining activity and eating healthily are described in the section on sport, physical activity, and diet in Chapter 6.

It can also be important to explain that side-effects are not static and immutable. Many, such as sedation, improve with time, and others can be helped by judicious dose adjustment or lifestyle interventions. It is important to give the young person information that certain side-effects are amenable to intervention.

A sense of the efficacy and utility of treatment is also necessary. As John McManamy (2007), an advocate for people with bipolar disorder, noted, "if people actually started feeling better on their meds they might turn out to be compliant" (p. 2). While somewhat cynical, this clearly highlights the subjective experience of a number of people with bipolar disorder, and the need for clinicians to ensure the best cost/benefit ratio for the young person.

Awareness of the importance of the therapeutic relationship and working collaboratively

The quality of the therapeutic alliance is a potent factor in determining adherence. Interpersonal and relationship factors, including trust and the level of involvement in decision-making, have been found to relate to medication adherence in people with physical health problems (Haynes, 1976), and seem likely to generalize to mental health difficulties.

In a review of the treatment alliance in bipolar disorder, Berk et al. (2004) noted that supporting client autonomy and self-efficacy may better promote medication adherence, as opposed to traditional models which emphasize the role of the clinician as the "expert." Berk et al. advocated an "enhanced autonomy" model, where informed decision-making is encouraged and the clinician's role is "not only as provider of information but also as facilitator of open dialogue" (p. 506), with this dialogue including discussion of medication side-effects. Similarly, Eisenthal et al. (1979) noted that what distinguished people who were adherent with their medication regimen from those who were not, was participation in treatment planning, and the clinician's understanding and assistance in meeting the client's requests. The move from a top-down concept of "compliance" to a collaborative model of "adherence" has in part resulted from recognition of the contribution that a sense of ownership of the treatment plan makes in adherence.

If able to do so genuinely, it can be effective to inform some young people that the clinician him/herself would take the medication, or would encourage a close family member to do so, if experiencing similar symptoms.

Providing honest and accurate psychoeducation

Psychoeducation regarding biological aspects of etiology and treatment, including benefits and side-effects of medication, can be extremely important. This can be particularly relevant when young people or their families have obtained inaccurate or misleading information regarding medication from the media or internet sites. Peet and Harvey (1991) found that providing psychoeducation – even when this included describing side-effects such as risks of toxicity – increased participants' knowledge about lithium and led to improved attitudes towards medication adherence. Psychoeducation can also involve informing the young person of the risks of non-adherence, which are described earlier in this chapter.

Psychoeducation can also be used to inform young people that while they may prefer to use "natural" medicines, there is a lack of direct evidence on the effectiveness of these, and they can also have side-effects. Individuals are encouraged to disclose the use of these medications to ensure the clinician does not prescribe any treatments that may interact.

Psychoeducation can also be used to address issues such as young people's beliefs that they will be more creative if becoming manic. For example, describing a "bell-curve" model of elevating mood can illustrate that medication can prevent the disorganization and lack of ability to create anything meaningful which can accompany severe mania.

Working with family members or significant others to encourage medication adherence

Evidence shows that people who have family support and supervision of medication have higher rates of adherence than those who do not (McEvoy et al., 1989). Therefore, it can be particularly important to be aware of each significant family member or friend's attitudes toward the young person taking medication, and to address any misconceptions. When family are involved in supervising medications, it can be important to help the young person negotiate how this will be done to minimize the chance of conflict.

Utilizing principles of motivational interviewing

Awareness of the motivational interviewing literature, and identifying the young person's "stage of change" regarding understanding of their disorder and medication adherence, can be valuable (see Chapter 8). This allows the clinician to design an intervention to assist medication adherence accordingly (Berk et al., 2004), and may be particularly helpful in young people who have a history of substance use.

Establishing routines and cues

If non-adherence occurs in the context of memory difficulties or disorganization, then routines and cues can be developed to assist with this. For example, the young person can be encouraged to establish a routine in which medication is always taken at a certain time, or a prompt is used, such as a regularly-timed television programme or brushing his/her teeth. Some young people report it being helpful to have their pills on a bedside table that is immediately visible when waking up or before turning off the light at night. Dosette boxes, or reminders programmed in a mobile phone, can also assist with memory-related adherence difficulties. Encouraging the young person to keep some medication in their wallet or bag can also reduce the chances of them missing doses if they are not at home at the time they usually take it.

Negotiating medication doses, "no medication," and "damage limitation"

When working with young people who are at high risk of non-adherence, it can be important to negotiate a compromise regarding medication. Specifically, attempting a trial of a reduced dose can be beneficial, as can undertaking a very slow reduction in medication, particularly if the young person agrees to more regular appointments and to allow the clinician to maintain contact with their family members, carers, or partner. While reducing medication may still result in the recurrence of symptoms, it can be important to trial this, to confirm that the clinician is hearing the young person's concerns. It may also allow the young person to experience the early phase of relapse in a relatively "safe" environment.

Similarly, discussion of a "no medication" option can enhance the therapeutic relationship and paradoxically lead to improved medication adherence in the longer term. While for most young people with bipolar disorder, not taking medication carries a considerable risk of relapse, it may be important for the clinician to discuss this as an option. Specifically, if a young person is adamant in refusing medication, for reasons such as certainty of not experiencing another relapse, the clinician can work collaboratively to design a behavioral experiment. This can include agreeing on what signs would be concerning to both the young person and therapist, monitoring these with family involvement if possible, and discussing what would constitute reasonable grounds to commence medication. The "contract" can also include the therapist requesting to see the young person more often if not on medication. Scott (2001) suggested that the most important aspect of this is establishing a clear agreement with the individual as to the circumstances in which the "experiment" would be deemed to have failed. Included in this would be agreement as to when the person would wish to "discontinue the no-medication trial," and how this situation would be managed. Scott also highlighted the importance of encouraging the client not to cease medication abruptly (to avoid rebound symptoms) but also that, if the person chooses to suddenly do this, they should feel able to tell the clinician so that both can accurately assess mental state.

In short, encouraging medication adherence in young people after only one or two episodes can be challenging, and is likely to require considerable negotiation, but if the clinician can maintain a good therapeutic relationship, the young person may be considerably less likely to experience a negative outcome.

Case study 4.1: medication attitudes matrix – Alan

Alan had been seeing his mental health team for around six months due to having experienced bipolar disorder with psychotic symptoms. He had made a good recovery, had been asymptomatic for around four months, and was considering stopping medication. Discussion between Alan and his clinician resulted in the matrix in Figure 4.1 being developed.

ADVANTAGES OF TAKING MEDICATION	ADVANTAGES OF NOT TAKING MEDICATION
• It makes me less speedy • It stops me doing stupid things (spending money and getting in fights) • It makes me less depressed • It allows me to keep going to college	• I don't need to remember to take pills when I see my mates or stay over at Dawn's (Alan's girlfriend) place • I can feel just like everyone else
DISADVANTAGES OF TAKING MEDICATION	DISADVANTAGES OF NOT TAKING MEDICATION
• It sometimes makes me feel like a "mental patient" • It makes me feel tired • I've put on weight	• I could get manic again • My parents and Dawn would get really angry and worried if I stopped

Figure 4.1 Medication attitudes matrix – Alan.

(A blank matrix is available in Appendix 6.)

Encouraging medication adherence when the person is asymptomatic

Because the risk of recurrence of bipolar disorder is lifelong for most individuals who have experienced significant symptoms, and due to evidence of the prophylactic effects of mood stabilizers, clinicians are often keen for people to continue taking these on an ongoing basis. However, a challenge is that this is an unpalatable message for most young people, and needs to be managed with great care to avoid alienation and disengagement. This can clearly be a significant challenge, as many young people, particularly after only having one episode, will raise the issue of discontinuing medication within weeks of remission of manic symptoms. Therefore, some young people believe that if their parents or clinician are encouraging them to keep taking medication, they must believe that they are still unwell. The following case study demonstrates one way in which this could be addressed.

Case study 4.2: encouraging prophylactic medication adherence – David

David was a 19-year-old man who initially presented with highly elevated mood, irritability, and grandiosity. His mood settled well on lithium, and David had reasonably good insight into having experienced a manic episode. This session occurred around two months after his initial presentation to our service.

DAVID: "You know how I've been going really well for a few weeks? I want to stop taking the lithium."

THERAPIST: "OK. Can you tell me how come?"

DAVID: "I just don't think I need it. Everyone says I'm going really well, and I don't think I need it any more."

THERAPIST: "I suppose that makes sense. You are going really well, and people only usually need medicine when they're sick. David, I guess

> though that one of the important differences between lithium and some other medicines is that it can work to make the manic symptoms go away, but can help keep them away too. Am I explaining that OK?"
>
> DAVID: "Yeah. Kind of."
>
> THERAPIST: "It's important that you know that we are not saying that you're sick. You're not. But we want to try to help you keep things that way. Some people take vitamin C tablets every day, not because they have a cold, but because they want to try to keep not having one. Does that make sense?"
>
> DAVID: "Yeah I suppose so, but I don't want to be on it for the rest of my life."
>
> THERAPIST: "I totally get that. How about we see how you go over the next few weeks and we'll keep it on the agenda to discuss. It might be that we can discuss a reduction in the meds with your doctor, but if I were to be totally honest, my advice would be that it would be good to take it for a while, and I'd give the same advice if you were my brother or a mate. It's also really important that you feel OK about letting me know if you're having any problems with it."
>
> DAVID: "Sounds OK."

Conclusions

- People diagnosed with bipolar disorder who are adherent with medication have better outcomes than those who are not.
- Medication adherence is poor amongst people with bipolar disorder in general, and poses an increased challenge for clinicians working with young people early in the course of the disorder.
- Stigma regarding having a mental health difficulty consistently emerges as a major reason for poor medication adherence in bipolar disorder. However, it is important for the clinician to anticipate and identify key reasons for non-adherence in each person they work with, and generate individualized solutions to this. This may involve practical suggestions (such as having a dosette box), motivational approaches, or other psychological interventions.
- Using multiple approaches – including maintaining a strong awareness of potential reasons for non-adherence, establishing a collaborative therapeutic relationship, regularly discussing benefits and side-effects of medication, providing psychoeducation, negotiating doses, and establishing practical plans including routines and cues – is likely to be the most effective way to increase medication adherence in bipolar disorder (Berk et al., 2004).
- Scott (2001) noted that patients rarely have medication adherence as a primary goal, and instead simply want to get relief from symptoms, return to their previous activities, and if possible, improve their sense of wellbeing. Therefore clinicians should ensure patients view medication as only one component in the treatment package. In addition, Scott asserted that if the medication regime is not acceptable, understandable, or manageable to the patient, then the clinician should not bother to supply the prescription as it is unlikely to be taken even as far as the pharmacy.

5 Cognitive behavioral therapy interventions

What we are today comes from our thoughts of yesterday, and our present thoughts build our life of tomorrow: Our life is the creation of our mind.

Buddha, in Haidt (2006, p. 23)

Introduction

As described in Chapter 1, a significant evidence base is emerging to support the application of CBT and other structured psychological interventions in the treatment of bipolar disorder. In a number of randomized controlled trials, CBT has been shown to decrease the duration of acute depressive episodes, extend the time between relapses, reduce hospitalization rates, and improve medication adherence and psychosocial functioning (for reviews see Huxley et al., 2000; Scott & Colom, 2005; Beynon et al., 2008). In addition, targeting prodromal cognitive changes, such as referential beliefs, has been found to increase the likelihood of successful outcomes in people with bipolar disorder (see review by Goldberg et al., 2005).

The focus of this chapter will be on the clinical application of selected cognitive behavioral techniques that we have noted to be particularly useful when working with young people with bipolar disorder.

CBT for young people with bipolar disorder: a phase-specific intervention

People require different elements of a cognitive behavioral intervention depending on their phase of the disorder. Specifically, in the acute phase, the emphasis tends to be on managing behavioral issues and risk reduction, including reducing stimuli if the person is manic or hypomanic, or increasing stimuli if depressed.

Later, during the early phase of recovery, the intervention can take a more cognitive focus, and may include the construction of a cognitive behavioral formulation. This will be collaboratively updated and elaborated during the course of the intervention. The early recovery phase also typically involves introduction to the theory and rationale behind the CBT model. This includes identifying and modifying unhelpful thinking styles and dysfunctional interpretations, whether these are excessively positive (during mania) or negative (during depression), and helping the person identify the impact of cognition on their disorder.

During the intermediate stages, work can include assessing the validity of unhelpful schemas, designing behavioral experiments, and utilizing other cognitive interventions to modify these.

The final stage focuses on relapse prevention and may include examination and modification of an individual's cognitive style or behavioral patterns, which may be specifically associated with their personal risk of relapse. This phase can also include identifying triggers and early-warning symptoms that allow the clinician and young person to intervene early before a full-blown bipolar episode develops.

The CBT model
Structure of sessions

Maintaining the focus of psychotherapy sessions can be challenging when working with young people who are manic, hypomanic, depressed, or experiencing a mixed episode. However, CBT may provide one of the most helpful psychotherapeutic models to assist the therapist with this, with a structure that encourages agenda-setting and regular summarizing, and concludes sessions with a brief review, preferably led by the patient. This can help to ensure that key elements have been retained by the young person, can assist correction of any misunderstandings, avoids miscommunication, and can allow collaborative reviewing of session goals. Some young people like to keep notes to consolidate work done in sessions, but this is not compulsory.

Reviews at around every six or seven weeks can be helpful, and allow the young person and the therapist to discuss progress. These reviews can enable the therapist to present visual feedback regarding change or progress in the form of graphs or scores from psychometric measures. Reviews also allow both the young person and the therapist to identify helpful and unhelpful aspects of therapy to date, and enable planning for future work. This structure can assist in developing a strong therapeutic relationship with young people with bipolar disorder through making it clear that the therapist wants to understand and include what is important for the young person.

A typical session would involve:
- Brief initial discussion as to how the person has been since the previous session.
- Asking the person what key elements they recall from the previous session (to allow for assessment of recall and address any misunderstandings).
- Checking previous homework if any was assigned.
- Collaboratively setting an agenda, generally consisting of two or three key items.
- Addressing agenda items.
- Summarizing the session (both therapist and client).
- Setting homework tasks.
- Arranging the next appointment.

In practice, adhering strictly to standard CBT protocols can be difficult, as attention and memory problems are common in people experiencing disordered mood. For this reason, when a young person is entering the early phase of recovery from mania or depression, it is even more important to recap and summarize regularly, and keep to simple goals. It may also be necessary for the clinician to take more of an active role in sessions during this time, and to have briefer sessions.

Introducing the CBT model

When starting therapeutic work, it can be valuable for the therapist to explain the rationale behind the CBT model, and how it can help the person with their experiences. This can include explaining the bidirectional relationship between thoughts, emotions, behavior, and biology, which can be done diagrammatically, utilizing Padesky and Mooney's (1990) model

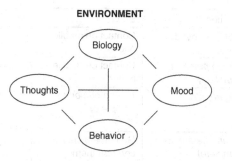

ENVIRONMENT

Figure 5.1 Diagrammatic CBT model. From Padesky and Mooney (1990). Reproduced with very kind permission of Christine Padesky.

(Figure 5.1). Rather than present the entire diagram initially, we find it useful to "build" it in stages on a whiteboard. For example, a common situation could be described in which a young person has the thought: "If I go to the party tonight, everyone will ignore me." The clinician can then demonstrate visually (by drawing an arrow from "thought" to "behavior") that this is likely to impact on the person's behavior, and result in him/her not attending the party. In turn, not attending, and therefore not testing the belief that no-one would talk to the person, could lead him/her to experience lowered mood, and contribute to further withdrawal and potentially even biological symptoms of depression. At this point arrows could be drawn connecting "behavior," "mood," and "biology." This in turn could lead to further withdrawal, lowered mood, and more unhelpful cognitions, demonstrated by arrows connecting "behaviour," "mood," and "thought."

We adapt this model for each person, depending on their presenting interests and mood, and ask the person to provide examples from their own experience of how their thoughts have impacted on their behavior and vice versa, how their behavior has impacted on their mood, and how these relate to biological aspects, with bidirectional links being made between each of the components of the model. We find that this model is generally easily comprehensible and helpful even for a young, first-episode bipolar population. The diagram can be referred back to during future sessions, acting as a simple cue to help clients remember the CBT model and understand their experiences within a CBT framework.

During the initial phase we also typically use another example to illustrate the relationship between cognitions, mood, and behavior. A situation is described where the person was supposed to meet friends at a particular venue on Friday night at 7 pm. It is 7.30 pm and no-one has arrived. The young person is asked for their initial automatic thought, which may be something like: "They are running late, because they've got held up in traffic." The person is then asked to describe how they might feel and how they would behave if they had this thought, which may be: "I would feel a bit annoyed, because I got there on time, and I might try to call them on their mobile phones." The person is then asked to list other potential automatic thoughts and describe the resultant mood and behavior. We then develop a grid which can be written on a whiteboard, with further examples, where "thought," "emotion," or "behaviour" is missing and the person is asked to complete the missing parts, with this illustrating the link between the three components (see Figure 5.2). Finally, the young person is asked to give their own example of a situation and describe the associated thought, emotion, and behavior.

Ensuring that the young person understands how interpretations of a situation can influence emotions and behavior can establish the foundations for future CBT work.

CBT formulation

While the clinician can begin developing an individualized CBT formulation on initial contact with the young person, or in some cases, even before this if clinical notes are available, it can be useful to construct this with the young person as their mood becomes more settled. If done collaboratively with the young person, constructing a formulation

Situation	Thought	Emotion	Behavior
Friends late	"They've got held up in traffic"	Mildly annoyed	Contact on mobile phone
	"I've got the wrong night/time/venue"	*(young person to complete)*	Contact on mobile phone
	"They have gone somewhere else without me"	Anger/sadness	*(young person to complete)*
	"They are bored with me/hate me/ are laughing at me"	*(young person to complete)*	Go home alone/ confront them
	(young person to complete)	Extreme anxiety	Contact friends' families/hospitals
	"They have set me up, and the authorities are on their way"	Anger/distress/ panic	*(young person to complete)*
	"I have a bit of time to myself"	*(young person to complete)*	Get a drink and relax
(Give own example of a situation and possible thoughts, emotions, and behavioral responses)	*(young person to complete)*	*(young person to complete)*	*(young person to complete)*

Figure 5.2 CBT grid.

can be extremely valuable, aiding initial engagement and the development of a therapeutic relationship in which the person feels understood by their therapist.

Typically, constructing a formulation involves assessing six key elements, which are:
- Significant experiences from the person's early history, including attachment issues.
- Core beliefs or schema.
- Conditional beliefs.
- Critical incidents in the person's life and their cognitive, behavioral, and affective impact.
- Factors that may maintain the disorder.
- Symptoms.
- Protective factors.

We will describe each of these in turn.

Early history and attachment

The first stage of developing a CBT formulation involves identifying key elements from the young person's early history, as described in Chapter 1. Particular focus on attachment issues can be valuable given their impact on mental health issues (see Chapter 2).

Schema

Beck et al. (1979) stated: "A schema constitutes the basis for screening out, differentiating, and coding the stimuli that confront the individual. He categorizes and evaluates his experiences through a matrix of schemas" (p. 13). Therefore, understanding and working with schemas is considered by many a central component of cognitive therapy, and comprises the second part of constructing a CBT formulation.

Jeffrey Young and colleagues have done considerable work in developing the understanding of schemas (Young & Klosko, 1993; Young et al., 2003; Young & Brown, 2005). While their focus has generally been on the relationship between schemas and personality disorders, we believe that schemas can also be influential in the development and maintenance of bipolar disorder. According to Young et al. (2003), schemas comprise not only the cognitions a person holds about themselves, the world, and the future, but also involve memories, emotions, and physical sensations. Schemas are described as unconditional, self-perpetuating, and fundamental to the person's sense of self.

There is evidence that schemas may have biological, genetic, and psychosocial origins, and that there may be bidirectional relationships between these. For example, LeDoux (1996) described an interesting interaction of nature and nurture, having found that traumatic events can organically alter the amygdala, which stores emotional memory, with this consequently impacting on further processing of information. Young et al. (2003) also noted that maladaptive schemas may result from "toxic childhood experiences" (p. 10), and that these subsequently influence the way a person views the world.

It can be particularly important to focus on schemas that may have impacted on the initial development of the disorder, act to maintain depressive or manic symptoms, or increase the young person's vulnerability to relapse. Discussion about life experiences, incidents, or situations which have been influential in the development of beliefs, or which have confirmed a particular schema, can be extremely valuable for both the therapist and the young person. For example, it may emerge that the young person started to notice their schema about failure in the context of regular humiliation by a parent, or that a specific traumatic incident or incidents were important in the formation of a schema relating to vulnerability or inability to cope. Exploration of the development of schemas can help the therapist develop empathy, understand how the young person sees the world, and appreciate how these beliefs originated, rather than simply viewing them as maladaptive cognitions that should be challenged.

When assessing young people with bipolar disorder, it is important not to assume their schemas based solely on their presenting symptoms at that point in time. Schwannauer (2003) noted: "It is therefore important to assess individuals' core beliefs independently of their presenting symptom pattern. A grandiose and manic individual might have the same core schema of 'unlovability' and 'incompetence' as a depressed person" (p. 262). Scott (2001) highlighted that in a manic phase, ideas about unlovability or incompetence can be redefined by the client with the common theme of "I'm different," which can then exacerbate grandiose or paranoid ideas that are a frequent feature of mania.

There are two further aspects of schema that are important to be mindful of during assessment. Firstly, schemas can be active or dormant. For example, a person may have abandonment schemas that are not evident while the person is in a relationship, but when the person is alone or a relationship has ended, they may experience significant distress. Similarly, a person may have perfectionistic schemas that are not problematic if the person always has time to prepare, but an urgent deadline which does not allow the person to complete the work to their satisfaction could be experienced as catastrophic.

Secondly, it may be important to note that schemas are not always pathological, and many can be quite adaptive. For example, perfectionism – described by Young and colleagues (2003) as "unrelenting standards" – manifested in schemas such as "things need to be in perfect order" or "I must do my best/can't settle for 'good enough'" will be rewarded in many environments. Similarly, self-sacrifice schemas such as "I need to put others' needs first" or "no matter how busy I am, I can always find time for others" may be common amongst healthcare workers. Difficulties only occur when the schemas are overly rigid or impact negatively on the person's life.

Young's maladaptive schema

The YSQ-L3 (Young & Brown, 2005) can be a very helpful tool in the assessment of schemas, with clinical observation and careful attention to recurring themes described by the person supplementing this.

Young has revised his schema work a number of times, but we recommend his recent book in collaboration with Klosko and Weishaar, *Schema Therapy: A Practitioner's Guide* (2003), which refers to 18 schema across 5 broad categories or "domains." While considerably more detail is provided in their book, the following is a brief overview.

Disconnection and rejection

Abandonment characterized by schemas such as "I worry that people I care about will leave me" or "people will always leave you in the end."

Defectiveness/shame characterized by schemas such as "I can't understand how anyone could love me" or "if people knew what I am really like, they couldn't care about me."

Mistrust/abuse characterized by schemas such as "people are rarely honest" or "people can't be trusted."

Emotional deprivation of nurturance, empathy, or protection, characterized by schemas such as "nobody has really been there for me."

Social isolation characterized by schemas such as "I feel isolated and alone" or "no-one really gets me."

Impaired autonomy and performance

Dependence/incompetence characterized by schemas such as "I need other people to help me get by."

Vulnerability to harm/illness characterized by schemas such as "I take great precautions to avoid getting sick or hurt" or "I feel that the world is a dangerous place."

Enmeshment/underdeveloped self involving extreme overinvolvement with others, characterized by schemas such as "I am so involved with my partner or parents that I do not really know who I am or what I want."

Failure regarding achievement, for example endorsing schemas such as "I often compare my accomplishments with others and feel they are much more successful."

Impaired limits

Entitlement/grandiosity characterized by schemas such as "I often get angry or irritable if I can't get what I want."

Insufficient control/self-discipline characterized by schemas such as "I often overdo things, even though I know they are bad for me."

Other directedness

Self-sacrifice where the person voluntarily helps others, often at their own expense. This is characterized by schemas such as "I feel very guilty if I let people down" or "If I do what I want, I feel very uncomfortable."

Subjugation where the person gives control to others due to feeling forced, or to avoid aggression, reprisals, or being rejected. This is characterized by schemas such as "I let other people have their way, because I fear the consequences" or "I will go to much greater lengths than most people to avoid confrontations."

Approval/recognition-seeking characterized by an excessive emphasis on approval, or where the person's sense of self-esteem is based primarily on the reactions of others. This would include endorsing schemas such as "it is important for me to be liked by almost everyone I know" or "I try hard to fit in."

Overvigilance and inhibition
Negativity/pessimism where the individual focuses on negative aspects of life, endorsing schemas such as "I often obsess over minor decisions, because the consequences of making a mistake seem so serious."
Unrelenting standards characterized by schemas such as "almost nothing I do is quite good enough; I can always do better."
Emotional inhibition characterized by schemas such as "I worry about losing control of my actions."
Punitiveness characterized by the belief that a person should be punished harshly for making mistakes, for example, believing "there is no excuse if I make a mistake."
Reproduced with very kind permission of Jeffrey Young

Conditional beliefs

The third element of constructing a CBT formulation is that of understanding the young person's conditional, or underlying, beliefs. Padesky (2000) has described conditional beliefs as "if . . . then . . ." phenomena. While many core beliefs or schemas originate during early childhood, it is typically not until later that conditional beliefs emerge. Awareness of conditional beliefs can allow the clinician a better understanding of the person's assumptions about his/her own role and its potential impact on events. For example, one person may express the core belief "the world is a tough place," but have the conditional assumption "but **if** I'm friendly, **then** others will be friendly back." However, another person may state: "The world is a tough place, so **if** I'm friendly, **then** others will take advantage of me." Clearly, understanding this additional information can allow the clinician a deeper understanding of the person's experience.

Conditional beliefs can be elaborated to inquire about the person's assumptions in relation to behavior, cognition, and mood. Asking the person to complete sentences such as "if I do . . .," "if I think . . .," and "if I feel . . ." can more clearly identify their conditional beliefs. For example, in response to these questions, one young person with whom we worked, who was prone to marked depressive episodes, stated: "If I'm not critical of myself, then I'm in danger of being lazy." This provided an excellent insight into his concerns about change and why previous therapy had been unsuccessful.

Critical incidents

The fourth aspect of constructing a cognitive behavioral formulation is that of assessing critical incidents in the person's life, and their affective, cognitive, and behavioral impact. While there can be some overlap with early history, critical incidents generally refer to events the person experiences in their teens and later, which significantly affect how the person sees the world or themselves, either by reinforcing existing schemas, significantly challenging these, or creating new core beliefs. For example, a serious assault could challenge a person's beliefs about the world being safe, whereas involuntary hospitalization could reinforce a person's pre-existing beliefs about being powerless or vulnerable.

Maintaining factors

The fifth aspect of the formulation involves understanding factors that maintain the person's cognitions, mood, and behavior. Maintaining factors can be situational, biological, behavioral, or cognitive. For example, remaining in an abusive relationship, or ongoing alcohol or illicit drug use, could maintain agitated or depressed mood. Increasing activity levels, risk-taking, and amphetamine use may increase excitability and manic symptoms.

Avoidance, whether behavioral (such as physically staying away from potentially difficult situations) or cognitive (such as attempting distraction from unpleasant thoughts), can be a powerful maintaining factor. This is particularly true in depression, as it is likely to result in the person not testing the validity of distorted beliefs.

Three common cognitive factors that may maintain manic or depressive symptoms are attentional bias, memory bias, and distorted interpretation of ambiguous information. Attentional bias refers to the tendency of people to attend to, and focus on, information that "fits" their current beliefs and mood, and discount information that does not. For example, when a person is manic or hypomanic, they may be more likely to attend to and recall perceived success, whereas when depressed the person may be more likely to focus on environmental cues that confirm their failures or negative beliefs. It can be important for the clinician to be aware of these attentional biases as they can powerfully reinforce and confirm the person's perceived appraisal of a situation or of him/herself.

The literature on autobiographical memory (e.g. Wessel et al., 2001; Peeters et al., 2002) has shown that, when depressed, people find it difficult to recall specific memories, either positive or negative, and instead tend to describe events in terms of general impressions. Mansell and Lam (2004) found that, similar to unipolar depression, people with remitted bipolar disorder were more likely to recall general rather than specific memories, particularly when this involved negative memories. The remitted bipolar group in Mansell and Lam's study also reported being able to recall more negative memories in everyday life than people with remitted unipolar depression. We find that young people often appear to find it difficult to recall positive experiences when depressed, whereas negative memories appear more easily accessible.

Memory bias can also include people "rewriting" their past, and reattributing positive or negative events. For example, when depressed, a young person could state "the only reason I was top of the class was because no-one else was really trying" or "he/she only said I did well to be nice." When manic or hypomanic, a person may reattribute criticism or negative appraisal by others as due to "jealousy." Similar to attentional bias, memory bias can be seen to maintain either mania or depression, as failures will be poorly recalled in mania, and successes forgotten in depression.

Distorted interpretation of ambiguous information involves processing "neutral" events – such as a person's facial expression or tone of voice – using biased explanations. For example, in psychotic mania, a person may feel that others are looking at him/her due to envy or because they are famous, whereas with delusional guilt that can accompany severe depression, a person may believe that the same facial expressions of others are indicative of anger or disgust.

It can also be particularly important for the clinician to assess social or environmental factors that may be maintaining symptoms. We have found that many young people with resistant depression describe situational factors that make change daunting (see case study of "Simon" later in this chapter), and impact on their motivation to attempt cognitive or behavioral techniques.

Symptoms

The penultimate element of the formulation is that of listing presenting symptoms under the headings: mood, cognition, and behavior.

Protective factors

The final part of the formulation is that of identifying strengths or protective factors. As noted in Chapter 2, mental health services often focus on pathology. However, acknowledging the young person's strengths can be an essential aspect of treatment, and may help encourage hope both for the clinician and the young person.

Case study 5.1: CBT formulation – Mohammed

Mohammed was an 18-year-old man of Lebanese Muslim background, living with his mother and 3 younger siblings. His father left home when Mohammed was aged 9, and was reported to have been very irritable and "religious" prior to this. Mohammed thought his father might have been "a bit crazy."

Mohammed's mother was often physically unwell when he was young, and he was often encouraged to be a "good boy" and look after his siblings. When Mohammed was 12, his mother experienced a complicated hysterectomy, which required him and his siblings to stay with his maternal aunt for around 2 months, during which he described feeling extremely lonely. His aunt could be quite strict and had high expectations of Mohammed's behavior.

Mohammed was an average student but was badly bullied at high school and reported feeling "stupid" and "different to everyone else." He left school aged 16, and commenced but failed to complete 2 apprenticeships. He thought he might have been depressed at this time, as he had felt significant sadness, was sleeping excessively, and had reduced his social contact.

Mohammed began to smoke around 2 grams of cannabis daily at the age of 15, but did not use any other illicit drugs.

He became more preoccupied with Islam after September 11, 2001, when he started to think he could be responsible for the "war" between Islam and the West.

Mohammed was admitted to an inpatient unit, as, for over 2 weeks, he had highly elevated mood, and was experiencing minimal sleep, impulsivity, and grandiose delusions about having a role in ending the "war." He had also been involved in a number of physical altercations with strangers due to trying to convert them to Islam. Mohammed also felt that he was able to communicate telepathically with world leaders. This had resulted from him noticing that politicians on television made statements on issues he had been thinking about, that they were wearing the same colour of clothing as him, and made gestures, such as nods, in a way that he felt indicated that they were saying: "Only you know what I really mean."

Prior to his manic episode, Mohammed reported having often felt depressed, occasionally experiencing suicidal ideation, and had recently reported that he may have to kill himself if he failed in his mission to keep his family safe.

The therapist worked with Mohammed to construct a diagrammatic formulation that made sense to him and included identifying Mohammed's strengths. The resulting diagrammatic formulation, which is a modified version of that described by Fennell (1989, p. 178), is shown in Figure 5.3, with a blank CBT formulation provided in Appendix 7.

The formulation letter

In addition to the diagrammatic CBT formulation presented in Figure 5.3, a formulation letter – commonly used in cognitive analytic therapy (Ryle & Kerr, 2002) – can be particularly useful. While there is not currently an evidence base for the use of such letters with young

Early history and attachment
Father experiencing mental health problems (genetic vulnerability?)
Father's religious beliefs
Father leaving home
Mother being unwell

|

Core beliefs/schema
People will leave me (**abandonment** – disconnection and rejection)
The world is dangerous (**vulnerability to harm/illness** – impaired autonomy)
I need to be responsible/good (**unrelenting standards** – overvigilance and inhibition)
I must put others' needs before my own (**self-sacrifice/subjugation** – other directedness)

|

Conditional beliefs
If I put my own needs first, I am being selfish
If I do things for others, they will like me/not blame me
If things go wrong, then it's my fault
If I worry, I'm a good person

Critical incidents	**Affective/cognitive impact**
Mother's hospitalization	Abandoned/people get ill/responsibility
Bullying at school	Different/vulnerable/alone/world a hard place
Didn't finish apprenticeships	Stupid/"a failure"
September 11	World dangerous/Islam versus "the West"

Maintaining factors
Cannabis use
Reduced social contact
Media coverage of issues around religion and terrorism
Cognitive factors (selective attention, interpreting ambiguous material)

Cognitions	**Mood**	**Behavior**
The world is at risk	Anxiety	Reduced social contact
It's my responsibility	Depression	Looking after others
I must be perfect	Guilt	
Others' needs come first	Fear	
Obsessional thoughts	Mania	
Confusion		

Protective factors
Strong social conscience
Strong work ethic
Likeable
Engaged with services

Figure 5.3 Mohammed's CBT formulation.

people with bipolar disorder, we believe they can give a valuable interpersonal framework for collaborative work.

The therapist would only write a formulation letter after considerable discussion with the young person, while the letter should clearly incorporate both parties' views and include agreement around key issues including treatment goals. Therefore, the letter should serve as a review of the sessions rather than present material to the person for the first time. There are a number of ways to write a formulation letter, which are likely to be heavily influenced by the degree to which the young person him/herself wishes to be involved, and may include the young person having the primary role in its construction.

Typically the formulation letter would:
- Describe possible underlying mechanisms and significant life events that may contribute to schemas, symptomatology, and presenting problems.
- Summarize key issues that have arisen in therapy to date.
- Identify future foci for therapeutic work.
- Highlight potential difficulties that may occur in therapy (both due to factors inherent to the young person, and those of the therapist).
- Suggest a collaboratively agreed problem list.

The following is an example of a formulation letter drawing from the previously described case of Mohammed (Figure 5.3). It should be noted that it was written in a style that the therapist felt was developmentally and intellectually appropriate for Mohammed, and reflected language that had been used during the sessions.

Dear Mohammed,
As we discussed, I wanted to write you a letter summarizing what I think has come up in our sessions so far. I've tried to cover all the main points we have talked about, but I'm really interested to discuss this with you and hear what you think.

When we first met, you were in hospital and it seemed that things were quite intense for you. You didn't want to be in hospital, and were confused as to why you had to stay there, which sounded really stressful, and maybe even a bit frightening.

However, during the first couple of times we met, you were able to tell me a few things about yourself and what it was like when you were growing up. I felt this was really important, because, as we discussed, sometimes things that happen to us when we are young can be really important in terms of how we feel about ourselves, and our thoughts and beliefs about other things later on.

For example, you told me that your dad had left home when you were young, and that you thought he might have been "a bit crazy." It sounds like after he left, you had quite a lot of responsibility and had to look after your brother and sisters, and that, in a way, you became the "man of the house." We talked about how it maybe felt quite good in some ways to have that responsibility, but that it also made you worry a bit too, and meant that it felt like sometimes you didn't really get looked after yourself. Another important thing you mentioned was that, a few years after your dad left, your mum got sick, and had to have an operation, and I wonder if this made you feel even more like it was your responsibility to take care of things and look after people, and also that if things went wrong, it felt like your fault.

Mohammed, we have talked a few times about how sometimes when people develop bipolar disorder and psychosis, the beliefs that they had before become stronger, and moods become more extreme, and I wonder if this is what happened with you. It seems it has always been important for you to look after your mum, brother, and sisters, but when you were in hospital, it felt like you had to look after the whole world, and instead of just putting your own needs on hold for a while, you felt like you actually had to die to be a good person.

As we have discussed, it seems possible that a number of things could have all contributed to you becoming really stressed, getting some of the thoughts and feelings you did, and going to hospital. We talked a bit already about how this can include biological causes, psychological causes, and stressful events. What I mean is, your dad having possibly had mental health problems, the fact you had a hard time at school, you being worried about the apprenticeships not working out, smoking cannabis, the thoughts that you had about people's safety, and hardly sleeping for almost a week all built up, with September 11 being the "final straw."

We talked a bit about how it might be good to spend some time in our sessions working on how we can keep getting things better for you, and to try to prevent your symptoms coming back. This could maybe include a combination of:

- Looking at how some of your thoughts might make you more at risk.
- Watching what stressful things happen in your life.
- Taking your medicine.
- Working out what your family could do that would be helpful.
- Helping you with your sleep.
- Cutting down or stopping cannabis.
- Helping you to start catching up with friends again.
- And as you said, maybe starting a course or job.

I think we have been able to work really well together so far, and I have been really impressed by how open and honest you have been with me about things that have happened in your life. But I wonder if, because you think a lot about looking after other people, it may be hard for you at times to ask me, or other people, for a bit of support when you need it. For me this would actually be a useful goal for us to work on, but I'm not sure what you think about this.

I look forward to hearing your thoughts about this letter and plans for our future work. Yours sincerely,

Cognitive and behavioral techniques for work with bipolar disorder

Earlier in this chapter, we described introducing the CBT model, development of a collaborative formulation, and assessment of schema. The following section addresses specific cognitive and behavioral techniques for working with young people with bipolar disorder.

We again highlight the importance of identifying maintaining factors, particularly of depressive symptoms, because if these are not addressed early in therapy, facilitating change can be difficult. This is illustrated in the following case study.

> ## Case study 5.2: working with social/environmental factors which maintain depressive symptoms – Simon
>
> Simon was a 20-year-old man who had been experiencing depressive symptoms characterized by anergia, anhedonia, and hopelessness for around 12 months following a brief manic episode. He had spoken with 2 previous therapists who had been unable to help him with this.
>
> An important part of the intervention with Simon in the first session was to identify his underlying concerns about change. He was therefore asked: "Simon, can you tell me what you are worried might be *worse* if you were no longer feeling depressed?" Although initially bemused, Simon was gradually able to acknowledge

that he had experienced significant pressure from his mother to find work since leaving school at 17, and this caused him considerable anxiety as he had struggled academically. Simon stated that since being diagnosed with depression, his mother no longer asked him to find work and had been more supportive of him. Later in the session, Simon also disclosed that his father had been quite physically aggressive towards him in the past, and his brother had been verbally critical towards him, with these also having stopped since Simon became depressed.

The therapist acknowledged that it was completely understandable that Simon would be extremely hesitant about anything which could improve his mood, and that there would need to be some extremely good reasons for him to "give up" his depression. Interestingly, Simon stated that he felt that his relationship with his father and brother was considerably improved, and that he felt there was significantly less likelihood that he would face further aggression from them.

Simon also requested that the therapist did not disclose too much detail with his family as his mood began to improve, until he recovered enough to work with the therapist on finding employment or a study course. The therapist agreed, with them having a shared joke that Simon could eventually "reveal" his recovery to the family in the style of a reality TV makeover show.

It was felt extremely important to identify any potential maintaining factors in the first session, prior to commencing any other CBT work. Describing the CBT model or recommending behavioral experiments without a clear understanding of Simon's family dynamics would have been unlikely to have been successful in this case.

Behavioral aspects of managing depressive episodes

A significant amount has been written on behavioral techniques for depression, and we recommend Scott (2001) and Blackburn and Davidson (1995) for further reading. However, we encourage the following:

- Activity scheduling, where tasks which the young person has previously found enjoyable or rewarding are deliberately undertaken, even if the person does not initially feel like doing so (see Appendix 8). However, it may be important to pre-empt with the young person that while they are initially unlikely to find these activities as enjoyable as previously, this should not be a deterrent from attempting them. We find that it is important for young people to achieve small goals early in therapy to encourage hope and self-efficacy. Taking the approach of "fake it 'til you make it" can be helpful, emphasizing that improvement often occurs in depression not by the person waiting to feel better before attempting tasks, but by undertaking behavioral tasks *despite* not feeling better, with cognitive and emotional change occurring *after* this. Johnson (1996) summarized this approach, stating: "Change the behavior; then the attitudes will change" (p. 369).
- Ensure that the young person avoids procrastination and attempts to "stay on top of" existing tasks or chores in order that they do not become overwhelmed and at risk of further depression or hopelessness. Encouraging the young person to recognize excuses for avoiding situations and to list these can be valuable. This strategy is illustrated in the case example of "Simone" in Chapter 9.
- Encourage the young person to remain engaged in social contact even if this feels difficult and is not as rewarding as when the person was not depressed. This can include assisting the person to plan activities that keep him/her in contact with friends but have relatively low social demands, for example, going to the cinema together.
- Risk assessment around self-harm and suicide should be undertaken.

Behavioral aspects of managing manic or hypomanic episodes

In relation to mania and hypomania, perhaps the most significant aspect of behavioral intervention in the early phase is encouraging reduction in the amount of stimulation the young person is experiencing. As Kahn (1990) noted, "the desired goal of individual or family psychotherapy in acute mania is not cure of the episode, which only time or medications will accomplish, but moderation of the most extreme manic behavior that can irreversibly devastate lives" (p. 234). Specifically, this can involve the following:

- Newman et al. (2002) described the "wait 48 hours before acting rule" (p. 62). This can include encouraging the young person to delay major life decisions, spending large sums of money, getting tattoos or piercings, or engaging in new sexual relationships.
- Linked to the intervention described above, Scott (2001) suggested that people can keep a "black book" and note their "good ideas" when manic or hypomanic. The rationale presented to the client is that once his/her mood is more settled and people appear to be taking him/her seriously again, the good ideas can then be selected and presented to people who may then be more receptive. Clients find this helpful as they feel the therapist is not dismissing every idea presented at this stage. Furthermore, the experience of re-reading these notes at a later date can be useful by promoting self-discovery of the fact that some of the ideas were truly irrational and could have had negative consequences had they acted on them immediately.
- Encourage the young person to avoid caffeine, alcohol, or illicit substances. High rates of caffeine consumption are common in people with mental health problems (Mester et al., 1995), but can be associated with increased levels of anxiety, physiological arousal, and impaired sleep. We have noticed that a number of young people consume significant amounts of energy drinks, particularly around times of increased study or social activity. However, the young person should also be discouraged from abrupt caffeine withdrawal, as this can result in lithium toxicity for some people (Mester et al., 1995). Therefore, any reduction in caffeine intake should be done gradually, with ongoing monitoring of lithium blood levels.
- Encourage the young person to avoid situations that could involve physical harm, such as extreme sports, sexual promiscuity, or driving.
- Discourage the young person from giving away any possessions or money until their mood is more settled.
- Construct a "decisional balance" of potential gain versus risk of behaviors. Newman et al. (2002) described working with the person to identify the "productive potential" versus the "destructive risk" of particular behaviors or activities (p. 58). Again, this may not stop the behavior in someone who is manic, but may allow for time to evaluate options.
- Activity priority forms can be developed, where the person is encouraged to list what needs to be done and how urgent each of these activities is. In practice this can be difficult to achieve when the young person is manic or hypomanic as they may view everything as equally important. However, attempts to prioritize activities can nevertheless be encouraged.
- Newman et al. (2002) advised encouraging the person to ask the opinions of at least two trusted others before commencing new projects or making important decisions (p. 57).
- Encourage the young person to actively seek situations which have been calming in the past, such as spending time with particular people, doing specific behaviors (such as having a bath, going for a walk, or listening to calming music), or being in familiar, low-stimulus environments. It can be helpful to design a list of these with the person when their mood is settled, and in consultation with family members.

- Family work can be particularly helpful for young people, where irritability may be more common than euphoria. This can focus on identifying situations that may exacerbate agitation, paying special attention to unhelpful communication styles (see Chapter 7).
- Encourage the young person to have more regular contact with his/her clinician, which can include daily telephone contact if necessary.

It should be noted that the strength of the therapeutic relationship is critical to the likelihood of the person being able to employ many of these behavioral strategies, as in a manic state, holding back from a desired activity may feel counter-intuitive and result in increased agitation. Furthermore, research has indicated that, when high mood is induced, people with bipolar disorder are significantly less likely to take advice (Mansell & Lam, 2006). However, the young person may be less likely to behave impulsively if discouraged from doing so by a trusted clinician or caring family member.

Mood monitoring

Mood diaries or records can take various forms, with some of those described in the literature involving considerable amounts of detail. As Goodwin and Jamison (1990) noted, mood recording "is useful not only in noticing patterns of mood and treatment response but also in giving patients a sense of control, instilling a feeling of collaborative effort, and underscoring the importance of systematic observation" (p. 735).

However, we have found that in practice, mood monitoring can be considerably more difficult with young people than is suggested in the literature, particularly as young people in the early stages of bipolar disorder are highly unlikely to complete rigorously detailed mood forms on a regular basis. In fact, in this population, people who do complete such forms may be at risk of overidentification with the disorder, may be driven by extreme anxiety, or may be overly concerned about pleasing the therapist.

There are a number of different ways of mood monitoring with young people. We generally use an abbreviated method in which we ask people to rate their mood on a 0–10 scale, with 0 indicating severe depression, or the worst the person has ever felt, 10 indicating extremely high mood, or the best they have ever felt, and 5 signifying the middle of the normal range. This is then plotted on a graph, with the young person and therapist collaboratively noting significant events that may have influenced mood (see Appendix 9).

However, young people often need significant assistance in defining anchor points for their mood and help understanding that it goes beyond a simple "happy versus sad" dichotomy. Helping the young person recognize that their mood is likely to be labile, and inclusion of monitoring irritability, can also be helpful. Scott (2001) noted that "happy" may be a misnomer (as dysphoria and mixed states are common in manic phases), and suggested two additional strategies. Firstly, the ratings can be of "depression" and "hyper" (or another term that captures what a "high" state looks like), and secondly that the ratings of hyper and depression can be made on separate scales. This allows for simultaneously high scores on ratings of both depression and mania (e.g. mania characterized by labile or mixed mood states) rather than forcing the young person to rate mania and depression as a dichotomy.

We also ask the young person to identify events, preoccupying thoughts, behaviors, or other contexts that may account for fluctuations in their mood, both retrospectively and for potential future events. It can also be valuable to spend time identifying potential stressors or events that could disrupt sleep, activity patterns, or medication adherence in the upcoming week. In terms of the "event-congruency hypothesis" (Francis-Raniere et al., 2006), described in Chapter 1, it may be helpful to establish which types of events may impact most notably on the person's dominant schemas and are therefore the most likely to precipitate changes in mood.

We find that this in-session approach to mood monitoring is more likely to promote regular self-monitoring, whilst reducing the anxiety that can be induced by excessive self-monitoring. It can also serve as an opportunity to reinforce the young person's understanding of the CBT model and the interrelationships between their thoughts, feelings, and behaviors.

Vicious cycles

Jones et al. (2002) described the role that vicious cycles play in the escalation of both manic and depressive symptoms. Specifically, when people are becoming hypomanic, they may feel more energetic, leading them to become increasingly excited that depressive symptoms have reduced. Consequently, the person may stay up later at night for work or social reasons, with this resulting in reduced sleep, seeking more stimulation, and having more energy, with symptoms gradually escalating towards mania.

In depression, initial anergia may result in withdrawal from social contact or other fulfilling activities, and lead to further hopelessness and increased anergia. In depression, "self-fulfilling prophecies" can also occur in which the person holds beliefs that they will fail or not enjoy a task, with this subsequently affecting their performance and resulting in these beliefs being validated. Furthermore, procrastination and avoidance due to initial lack of energy in depression can lead to increased anxiety at leaving tasks incomplete, which then exacerbates low mood and may lead to an increased sense of hopelessness.

It can be helpful to work with people to identify their specific idiosyncratic cycles early, and attempt to pre-empt these before they become apparent. To manage this, the therapist can encourage the setting of small goals, which can be completed as homework. It appears very important, however, that such goals are attainable, to avoid a further sense of failure. This is discussed in the next section.

Goal setting and homework

The setting of homework assignments is recognized as an important component of many CBT manuals for mood and psychotic disorders (Beck et al., 1979; Chadwick et al., 1996; Ramirez-Basco & Rush, 1996), but it is only in recent years that an evidence base has begun to accumulate showing its efficacy. One of the largest studies to examine the effectiveness of homework involved a meta-analysis of 27 studies, with a total of 1702 participants (Kazantzis et al., 2000). Results showed that psychological therapy which included homework assignments was correlated with a significantly better therapeutic outcome than therapy which did not include homework.

Similarly, a recent paper by Rees et al. (2005) indicated that for people with either depression or an anxiety disorder, the quality and quantity of completed homework predicted outcome in terms of symptom measures and quality of life. Furthermore, they found that while cognitive tasks such as thought records were more influential in reducing anxiety scores, behavioral homework tasks such as scheduling pleasant activities and exposure were the most important predictors of reduced depression and improved quality of life. Interestingly, no correlation was found between severity of symptoms and likelihood of homework completion. This would indicate that it was not simply people with less serious symptoms who were more likely to complete homework and therefore experienced better outcome.

We find that some modification is necessary when setting homework tasks for a young population that is early in the course of bipolar disorder. Specifically, as described in Chapters 2 and 3, insight and engagement difficulties can mean that setting excessive homework without a solid therapeutic relationship or shared agenda is unlikely to be successful. Instead, a more Socratic approach may be required in which the young person is asked to identify what *they* think they could try between sessions which could help them, and why they think it will work. We have found that this can often result in some unexpected and imaginative answers, particularly as the young person has access to information about their lives and circumstances that the therapist does not.

We also recommend that it can be valuable for the therapist to play "devil's advocate" after the young person has suggested a homework activity. This can include asking clarifying questions such as "how do you think doing . . . will help?" or "can you explain to me what it is about trying . . . that is going to make things better for you?" This can help to ensure that the young person is not simply stating what they think the therapist wants to hear, and can enhance motivation to try the homework task.

A further important consideration when setting homework tasks for young people with bipolar disorder is that they may require more planning. Specifically, distractibility, poor concentration, disorganization, or amotivation may mean that the therapist needs to take more time, not only to clarify the objective and purpose of the task, but also to design a more "step-by-step" approach. As noted in the literature on homework in psychotic disorders, people are more likely to complete homework if they clearly understand the rationale behind it (Glaser et al., 2000). Exploration of potential barriers to homework completion and generating potential solutions to these can also be important.

As mentioned earlier regarding mood monitoring sheets, we generally find that young people are not keen to complete excessive written homework, and young men in particular are more likely to attempt homework that is more practical or activity-based. This can include activity scheduling to assist with mood difficulties (see pp. 77, 102, and 157), or undertaking behavioral tasks, such as graded exposure to manage comorbid anxiety difficulties or reduction of substance or alcohol use. Homework which we find helpful for young people with bipolar disorder can also include interpersonal assignments such as testing out assertiveness skills or attempting different communication styles with friends, school or work colleagues, partners, or family members.

It is also important when setting homework that the tasks are clear and have a high likelihood of success, particularly if the young person is vulnerable to low self-esteem or self-criticism. We have found that in the early phase of recovery from depression, young people will often paradoxically set themselves excessively challenging tasks, such as expecting themselves to be able to attend the gym every morning after a significant period of not exercising, or expect to alter a reversed sleep-wake cycle in two or three days. This is consistent with the finding by Johnson (2005), noted in Chapter 1, that people with bipolar disorder tend to set themselves challenging tasks and goals. Unfortunately, when depressed, people often lack the motivation to be able to achieve these goals. In addition, and in direct contrast to when manic, any successes are commonly minimized, leading to less incentive to pursue further goals. The result is the "worst of both worlds," in which the person may feel hopeless, but still expects him/herself to be able to meet what may be unreasonable self-imposed objectives, with the resulting failure to do so leading to further hopelessness and self-blame. If left unchecked by the therapist, an unsuccessful homework task is likely to lead to an increased sense of hopelessness, and can be damaging to the therapy.

In order to avoid this further downward spiral of hopelessness and diminished motivation, we feel it is essential for the clinician to carefully monitor homework tasks, ensuring that they are at a level in which the person is likely to be successful, but are not so undemanding that they are pointless. Glaser et al. (2000) recommended that before collaboratively setting any homework task, clinicians should ensure that patients have a confidence level of 70% or above in being able to complete it. While this appears reasonable, clinicians working with young people with bipolar disorder should take into account the potential impact of ongoing mood symptoms when collaborating on homework. Specifically, overconfidence when hypomanic, or underconfidence when dysphoric or depressed, may impact on the appropriateness of the homework task suggested by the young person.

A significant risk when setting small, achievable goals is that achieving these is likely to be minimized by the person when depressed. It is therefore important that the clinician helps the person keep the "bigger picture" goal in sight, by clearly emphasizing that each of the steps towards this is valuable in itself. The analogy of an athlete recovering from a sports injury can be useful in this regard, with encouragement that while the person's objective is still attainable, progress should be gradual, and setting excessive targets too early is counter-productive and may in fact lead to setbacks.

Finally, there is evidence that the likelihood of homework being completed is at least partially determined by the response of the clinician and the seriousness with which he/she appears to take it (Garland & Scott, 2002). Therefore, it is important that the clinician takes time at the start of each session to ask about how the previous homework task went. This can include identifying any difficulties encountered, giving feedback, and rewarding attempts made, even if unsuccessful, while attempting to instill internal reinforcement and a feeling of accomplishment in the young person him/herself.

Cognitive aspects of managing mania and depression

Cognitive therapy is built on the concept that there is an interrelationship between a person's thoughts, emotions, and behavior, and that working to develop more helpful cognitions and behavior can have an impact on a person's mood (see Padesky & Mooney, 1990, and Figure 5.1).

Both mania and depression are typically associated with thinking patterns that may be polarized (either positive or negative), flawed, or unhelpful, or maintain the person's mood state. One of the tasks for the therapist is to help the young person with bipolar disorder to identify and "catch" unhelpful, destructive, or inaccurate cognitions, and to assist in modifying these. In reality, whilst thought exploration can be undertaken in depression and to a reasonable level in hypomania, in mania the task is more likely to encompass a more simplistic exercise until the individual's mental state begins to stabilize. Initially, therefore, interventions for mania tend to focus on behavioral strategies that reduce the likelihood of acting on any ideas, particularly when these involve risk. However, this can be difficult, and therefore – if able to engage with and attend to the process – the clinician can encourage the young person to compare the perceived "gains or constructive" aspects of ideas with the potentially more likely "losses or destructive" outcomes (Scott, 2001).

Typical unhelpful or inaccurate thinking patterns include:

- **Overgeneralization** – where a single or limited number of events are viewed globally, e.g.
  "I failed that exam. I'm totally useless" (depressive).
  "I passed that exam. That means I'm a genius" (manic).
- **Dichotomous (all or nothing) thinking** – where the person views themselves or a situation in a completely polarized way, e.g.
  "If I can't be perfect, there's no point in trying" (depressive).
  "I'm the most amazing person in the world" (manic).
- **Personalization** – where a person views the outcome of a situation as solely due to their own influence, e.g.
  "Our team lost because I'm useless" (depressive).
  "Our school got good overall exam grades because I influenced everyone to do well" (manic).
- **Emotional reasoning** – where, because the person feels a particular way, it must be true, e.g.
  "I feel like a loser, so I know it's true" (depressive).
  "I'm the best fighter in the world because I feel really strong" (manic).
- **Selective abstraction** – where one piece of information is taken as evidence for the whole situation, e.g.
  "That guy at work criticized me. They all think I'm crap at my job" (depressive).
  "I won that race at school so I'm the fastest person in the world" (manic).
- **Arbitrary inference** – where the person "jumps to a conclusion" with little or no evidence, e.g.
  "My girlfriend seemed weird today. She's going to finish with me" (depressive).
  "That girl stared at me because she knows I'm a legend" (manic).
- **Magnification or minimization** – where the person exaggerates negative aspects of a situation and ignores positive ones, or vice versa, e.g.
  "The coach criticized my defence during the game. He thinks I'm useless" (depressive).
  "That teacher said he liked my essay. That proves I'm a genius" (manic).
- **Fortune-telling** – where a person believes they can tell the future, e.g.
  "I'm going to get shouted at by my boss" (depressive).
  "I know that everyone will love me at the party" (manic).
  N.B. "Fortune-telling" can sometimes lead to a self-fulfilling prophecy. For example, believing that he/she will fail an exam may lead to a person experiencing increased anxiety, inability to study, and poor sleep, and result in poor performance.
- **Attentional bias** – where the person focuses only on events which "fit" with their current mood, e.g.
  "That person looked at me because they know I've got a mental illness" (depressed).
  "That guy talked to me on the train because he knows I'm an amazing dancer" (manic).
- **Memory bias** – this is described above (p. 10–11 and 72) and refers to a cognitive style in which the person's mood influences the information from their past which is recalled, e.g.
  "I always screw up. I can't remember any good things I've done" (depressed).
  "I'm amazing. When I look back, everything I've done has been sensational" (manic).
- **Self demands** – in depression, people often describe their negative thoughts as being characterized by **"shoulds," "musts,"** or **"have tos."** For example, people will report that they believe they *must* do well all the time, *should* come top of their class, or *have to* be liked by everyone.
- **Thoughts relating to fear of mania** – we find that a number of young people who have experienced a manic episode report automatic thoughts relating to fear of manic relapse. Specifically, some young people report a fear of becoming "too happy," or of doing anything too exciting, and will consciously "rein themselves in" when experiencing even normal periods of improved mood.

Socratic questioning

The Socratic method is consistently cited as an important technique in cognitive therapy, but is often not well defined (Overholser, 1993). However, in one of the most informative clinical papers describing Socratic questioning, Padesky (1993) identified four main components.

The first aspect is that of "asking information questions" (p. 17), where the therapist takes time to clarify clients' concerns. In cognitive therapy for depression, this could involve asking the person to be clear what they mean when they describe themselves as "a loser" or "a failure," rather than assuming the person's definition and proceeding to "challenge" this prematurely. This stage can also involve establishing how the person's beliefs may have originated, including identifying events or individuals that have been important in the formation of their beliefs (described in the section on schema assessment in Chapter 2). When doing this, the therapist needs to be prepared for the emergence of information which may fit with the young person's beliefs, and for the young person to describe events in which they have in fact experienced failure or been told they are "a loser." Socratic questioning encourages the therapist to accept that the person may be correct in their beliefs, and that it is not necessarily the therapist's task to prove these beliefs wrong.

The second element of Socratic questioning described by Padesky (1993) is "listening" (p. 17), where the therapist is not simply attempting to accumulate evidence to change the person's mind, but is willing to receive unexpected answers to their questions. Listening to the young person can also be particularly rewarding as it allows for identification of solutions that the therapist may not have considered. O'Hanlon and Weiner-Davis (1989) suggested: "Our clients perpetually teach us how to work with them, to help solve their dilemmas" (p. 8).

The third phase of Socratic questioning involves "summarizing" (p. 18), which Padesky (1993) suggested should occur every few minutes, allowing the therapist to clarify that they understand the young person correctly, and ensuring that the young person understands the therapist.

The final element of Socratic questioning involves "synthesizing and analytical questions" (p. 19), which Padesky (1993) suggested is unfortunately often omitted by therapists, despite being of critical importance. This involves the therapist asking the young person how information that has emerged during the session has been integrated, for example by inquiring: "How does what you have just said fit with the idea that you're a loser?"

Socratic questions

We have found that a number of questions can be helpful as part of a Socratic intervention, including:

- How long have you believed/felt that . . .?
- What did you think before . . .?
- What made you first think/feel that . . .?
- How did you come to believe/feel that . . .?
- How sure/convinced are you that . . .?
- What makes you so sure that . . .?
- Are there times that you have had doubts about . . .?
- What does your friend/mother/father/brother/sister/girlfriend/boyfriend think . . .?
- What doesn't make sense to you about . . .?
- What doesn't fit about . . .?
- Is there any evidence that . . . isn't the case?

- What other explanations could there be for . . .?
- What else could be going on?
- What would need to happen for you to doubt . . .?
- What would it mean if . . . was true?
- What would it mean if . . . wasn't true?
- What are the advantages of believing that . . .?
- What are the disadvantages of believing that . . .?
- What is helpful about thinking that . . .?
- What is unhelpful about thinking that . . .?
- How could we test out if . . . is true?
- What would you say to someone else who told you this?

Considering alternatives: the "responsibility pie"

People may be more likely to jump to conclusions, or to only consider extremely limited options, when either manic or depressed. Therefore, perhaps one of the most effective techniques of cognitive therapy is to encourage the young person to view their thoughts as *hypotheses*, which might or might not be true. While agreeing that the person's thoughts or beliefs may make sense in terms of their life experience, the clinician can help the young person understand that these can change and may not be true for all situations, and that other factors may be contributing to the situation. Jones et al. (2002) described using pie charts to manage rigid beliefs, where the clinician and client work collaboratively to identify *all* possible explanations for an event and the percentage likelihood of each. This is then represented diagrammatically. The following case study describes this process.

Case study 5.3: responsibility pie – George

George was a 21-year-old man diagnosed with bipolar disorder who was vulnerable to low mood in the context of extreme self-criticism. George described ongoing low mood, stating that he felt extremely guilty that his friend John had used cannabis for the first time at a party they both attended. George felt solely responsible as he had used cannabis on a number of occasions in front of John, and had occasionally offered joints to John in the past.

The therapist identified one of the central cognitions, which appeared to drive George's guilt, and asked George to rate the strength of this belief and the associated affect, which were as follows:

INITIAL BELIEF	STRENGTH OF BELIEF	ASSOCIATED AFFECT
"I am totally to blame for John starting to smoke cannabis"	100%	Guilt 90% Sadness 50% Anxiety 20%

Cognitive therapy focused on assisting George to examine other possibilities as to why John had used cannabis on that occasion. This was done through asking Socratic questions such as:

"I'm interested as to what was happening when *you* first used cannabis, George. What do you think were the reasons for you?"

"Who else was there with you?"

"Had John ever talked about smoking cannabis before?"

"What kind of pressure was on John to use cannabis from other people?"

"What else was going on to make John smoke that night?"

"What did John actually say to you after you both smoked?"

"Who was it that 'made' you smoke cannabis the first time?"

George was gradually able to identify that a number of factors had contributed to John using cannabis at the party. He was then asked to estimate the percentage influence he believed each of these had contributed to John's cannabis use. These included John's own wishes and previously expressed interest in trying cannabis (10%), the fact he had just been paid (20%), an argument John had with his girlfriend, Mel (20%), that another friend, Ally, was also there but didn't stop John smoking (20%), in addition to George's influence (30%).

This was illustrated visually in Figure 5.4.

Following this exercise, George described two modified beliefs, which led to significantly less conviction in his personal responsibility and an associated reduction in negative affect.

REVISED BELIEFS	STRENGTH OF BELIEF	ASSOCIATED AFFECT
"Although I was partly to blame, there were lots of things that contributed"	70%	Guilt 20% Sadness 5%
"John's a big boy, and while I might have had an influence, he kind of wanted to do it too"	30%	Anxiety 1%

Figure 5.4 George's responsibility pie.

(A blank "responsibility pie" is available in Appendix 10.)

Finding alternative explanations to the person's unhelpful thoughts is important, but these have to be acceptable to the person. When a person is depressed it is unlikely that their cognitions will change rapidly from "I'm a total failure" to "I'm a total success and everyone loves me," unless becoming manic. What appears more likely is a believable counter-argument such as: "Like everyone else, there are some things I'm bad at and some I'm good at." Mooney and Padesky (2000) suggested it is important for the person to develop these in their own words, as the new beliefs may not necessarily be the linguistic opposite of the previous ones.

Beliefs and meaning

A recent development in cognitive therapy has suggested that people's cognitions contain two qualitatively different levels of meaning, namely "propositional" and "implicational" meaning (Teasdale & Barnard, 1993; Gumley et al., 1999). Propositional meaning refers to whether a piece of information is actually true or not, whereas implicational meaning refers to what it *means* to the person if the information is true or not. For example, a young man may experience the thought that he is gay, which may cause him distress. Traditional cognitive therapy may have focused on working with propositional meaning, that is, whether it is true that he is gay, by examining evidence regarding whether he had experienced a sexual relationship with another man, or had fantasized about gay sex. However, what may be more important and valuable in reducing the young man's distress is examining what it actually means for him if others think he is gay, and possibly working on unhelpful or inaccurate stereotypes he may hold about homosexuality.

Case study 5.4: implicational meaning and grandiose delusions – Vu

Vu was a 20-year-old man of Vietnamese background who had migrated to Australia with his family at the age of 14. He was living in run-down rented accommodation and was inactive for much of the day. He had attempted some part-time work but found this difficult due to having a reversed sleep cycle. He had developed a clear manic episode, and previously presented as elevated and agitated, with pressured speech, flight of ideas, and grandiose beliefs. Vu had some ongoing hypomanic symptoms at the time of the session.

THERAPIST: "How have things been going?" (*Leading with open question, as agenda not clear.*)

VU: "OK. But I still keep thinking a lot about whether I'm famous or not."

THERAPIST: "Is that a problem for you?" (*Clarifying whether this should be a target for further work.*)

VU: "Well, you know, it's just annoying. I'm just not sure, and it annoys me sometimes. Because I still get a bit freaked out by people looking at me."

THERAPIST: "What are you thinking you might be famous for?"

VU: "I used to think I'm an actor. But I don't think so. I think it might be a reality TV thing, you know?"

THERAPIST: "What kind of things have happened that have made you think you might be famous?" (*Examining evidence involved in the development and maintenance of the belief.*)

VU: "Just when I walk down the street. People look at me and notice me. And they look at me like they know that I'm famous."

THERAPIST (*looking for additional evidence supporting the belief*): "Are there other things that make you think you're famous?"

VU: "No. It's mainly that."

THERAPIST: "What would it feel like if you *were* famous?" (*Attempting to identify the implicational meaning of the belief for Vu.*)

VU (*PAUSE*): "I'd be doing something with my life."

THERAPIST (*clarifying the specific meaning of this*): "What do you mean?"

VU: "I'd have a girlfriend who would call me and we would go out to eat. And I'd have a job I was important at."

THERAPIST: "That sounds alright. Anything else?"

VU: "I could go fishing at the weekend and read a book every night. Maybe have coffee with friends . . . and I'd hardly watch TV."

THERAPIST: "Sounds pretty good."

VU: "Sometimes I think I might just imagine being famous."

THERAPIST: "Hmmm. What makes you think that?"

VU: "Well you've seen my house and it's pretty crap. And it's a mess. And I just do the same boring things every day."

THERAPIST: "Uh-huh. So what are you thinking?" (*Synthesizing question.*)

VU: "Well maybe my mind makes me feel famous, because it feels good when I feel famous. And I get more confident."

THERAPIST: "That would make a lot of sense. Are you saying that because things don't feel so great for you at the moment, sometimes it would be really nice to feel famous?" (*Summarising question.*)

VU: "That's it."

THERAPIST: "Vu, I was wondering. Can you think of a way we can work on you feeling better about yourself at the moment, and doing some of the things you suggested, while we figure out the whole famous thing?"

In the above case, traditional cognitive therapy might have focused on gathering evidence as to the legitimacy of Vu's claim, such as asking him to record each time he appeared on television or in newspapers, or undertaking behavioral experiments such as picking random people in the street and asking if they recognized him from any media. This "rational" challenging of Vu's delusion would have been relatively easy, but it appears unlikely that it would have resulted in a positive outcome. In fact, even if "successful" in reducing the conviction of Vu's beliefs, it may have led to an increase in his depressive symptoms. Instead, however, the therapist asked Vu *what it would mean* if he were famous. Vu's answer not only clarified a potential function of his beliefs when elevated, but also informed the therapist of potential foci for future therapy, such as working on his social contact, employment, and increasing pleasurable activities.

Understanding the meaning of beliefs can be equally applicable for self-critical cognitions in depression. While such cognitions may appear purely unhelpful from the therapist's point of view, the young person may be very reluctant to give these up as he/she may feel that they are protective against laziness and help the young person maintain his/her high level of performance. Again, challenging on a solely logical or intellectual level is unlikely to be successful.

We therefore strongly recommend identifying the potential function of beliefs, whether apparently positive or negative, and clarifying the implications of change before beginning any cognitive intervention. As mentioned in Chapter 2, a clear psychological formulation can assist greatly with this.

Schema work in bipolar disorder

As discussed in Chapter 2 and earlier in this chapter, schemas are stable and enduring beliefs that develop during childhood and are considered to play an important role in a person's experience of the world. Schemas serve to filter our experience by influencing what we attend to, ignore, and recall. In both mania and depression, a number of influential schemas may be active, which will focus the person's thoughts on particular aspects of their environment, such as perceived inadequacies and failures when depressed, and success and infallibility when manic or hypomanic.

Schemas may impact on both the course of the disorder and its treatment, and Ball et al. (2003) suggested that when working with individuals with bipolar disorder it is important to identify schemas which increase their vulnerability to depression or mania. Specifically, they suggested that "core beliefs associated with the need for approval, worth based on achievement, defectiveness/failure, alienation, and trustworthiness of others" (p. 46) are important in this respect. Similarly, perfectionistic schemas are likely to impact on engagement and medication adherence, specifically if characterized by beliefs such as "I should be able to manage my moods without medication." Therefore, schemas can be an essential target for intervention with young people with bipolar disorder.

Modifying schemas

While a full description of schema therapy is beyond the scope of this book, we strongly recommend two books by Jeffrey Young and colleagues, *Schema Therapy: A Practitioner's Guide* (2003) and *Reinventing Your Life* (1993). The following describes some aspects of modifying schemas, which may be useful in work with young people with first-episode bipolar disorder.

Techniques to help modify schemas

- A significant initial aspect of schema work involves examining with the young person how their schemas may have originated, and then reframing the experiences from which the schemas were formed. Young et al. (2003) have provided a summary for therapists of the possible origins of each of the 18 schemas that were described earlier in this chapter. In helping young people to identify the origins of their schemas it can be useful to ask them to recall as many specific examples, images, or events as possible which relate to particular schemas about themselves, others, and the world. This can be important, as many young people will not have considered how their schema originated, and simply take them as "just how I am/people are/the world is."

  Highlighting that the source of a schema may have been a parent or significant other person making statements such as "you're not good enough," "it's a dog-eat-dog world," or "you need to do your best all of the time" can be valuable. Specifically, it can allow the young person to consider that the statement was the opinion of an individual rather than a fact, and may therefore be more open to challenge.

- After establishing the connection between schemas and early childhood experiences, it can be helpful to inquire about current relationships or recent incidents that may have maintained these beliefs. This can increase the person's awareness of how schemas are played out in their current relationships, including the therapeutic relationship.

- It can be valuable to identify and "catch" live examples of the young person's thinking patterns during sessions. Family sessions can also provide interesting insights into the intergenerational nature of some schemas, with parents or siblings often reporting similar thinking styles. Work on this can be done playfully, where, as homework, the young person has to notice and record every time their family member voices the specific unhelpful cognition, such as making a "should," "must," or "have to" statement, while family members are encouraged to do the same with the young person.

- It can be important to identify and illustrate the impact of attentional biases on a person's mood. A useful example can be pointing out that in the same way that we are much more aware of red traffic lights when in a hurry, people focus on failures when depressed, or successes when manic. Helping people find balance in this and to recognize alternative explanations to their initial overly positive or negative appraisals can be valuable in reducing the impact of the belief on mood.

- Young et al. (2003) described that one of the most important techniques of schema therapy is that of "empathic confrontation" (p. 47). This involves the therapist spending time reflecting with the person how the development of their schemas may be understandable given their life history, but also reflecting that these schemas may not be accurate or helpful.

  Specifically, if the schema relates to a belief voiced by a particular influential person, examining the "credentials" or authority of the person making the statement can be powerful. For example, it may help the young person to understand that the view voiced by the influential person that became the basis of the schema may be understandable in terms of that person's life experience, but may not be as applicable to the young person him/herself. When this specifically involves a critical comment made towards the young person, it can be valuable to help them understand that the person voicing this belief may have experienced significant criticism themselves or had an attachment history in which support or sensitivity were not modeled.

- On some occasions, rather than attempting dramatic changes to schemas, helping young people modify unhelpful aspects of these can be important. For example, as noted by Scott (2001) in the chapter on adherence, perfectionistic schemas such as "I should try harder" can impact negatively on medication adherence. However, this can be reframed as "I should try harder to get into a regular routine, remember to take meds, be less critical of myself, and attend appointments."

- Helping the young person take a historical approach can be valuable. Adopting a "that was then, this is now" approach can help the young person recognize that while it may have been helpful to hold a particular belief in the past, he/she does not need to accept it unconditionally now. Instead, the young person is encouraged to consider whether it is a useful way of viewing a current situation or whether there could be alternative views that are more adaptive or appropriate.

- In working with schemas, it is important that both the therapist and young person recognize the difficulty of change. Schemas often emerge to protect the person, and are likely to have served a function, at least in the past. Young (unpublished lecture, 2006) referred to schemas "fighting for their survival," and that "schema chemistry" can keep people entrenched in relationships or patterns of behavior, which, although unhelpful, nonetheless feel "right" to the person. Modifying existing schemas, even if logically more helpful to the person, can initially feel challenging and uncomfortable.

- It can be valuable to prepare the young person for the likelihood that they will initially discount evidence that does not "fit" with their schemas. Gentle humour can be used, with the therapist "predicting with a crystal ball" that the young person will initially ignore or challenge any new ideas.

- We sometimes encourage young people to view work on developing new schemas as similar to learning a new language. This can be particularly helpful when past attempts to change beliefs have been unsuccessful. The analogy of learning a new language acknowledges that the person's "default" state is likely to remain that of experiencing the previous depressed or dysthymic cognitions, at least initially. However, with practice, work on the new beliefs will begin to feel more natural and the young person will become more confident using them.

- Mooney and Padesky (2000) urged patience, but also encouraged optimism for therapists undertaking the process of change. They noted: "Clients who experience recurrent problems generally have spent a great deal of time, emotional energy, and physical effort trying to change how they feel and experience their lives . . . However, reliance on our client's creativity and tolerance of ambiguity and doubt are central to the therapeutic process we propose" (p. 151).

- Because people vulnerable to low mood can at times have highly critical self-schemas that may maintain this, Gilbert (2000) described the idea of "compassionate challenging." This involves the individual gently applying traditional cognitive therapy techniques to themselves. Gilbert encouraged patients "to try to challenge with as much warmth and understanding as you can manage. Your challenges should not be cold, bullying, or irritable in their emotional tone. The more you learn to have sympathy with yourself while at the same time looking for rational alternatives, the easier you may find it to change your feelings" (p. 349). This can include asking the person how they would respond to a friend who made a similar self-critical statement, or asking the person how they would like someone else to treat them when they think or feel negatively or self-critically.

- Padesky and her colleagues recommended that rather than simply challenging existing unhelpful schemas, it can be more fruitful to work with the person to construct new, more adaptive schemas, and to develop the evidence which supports these (Padesky 1994; Mooney & Padesky, 2000). They suggested that this focus could increase motivation, encourage collaboration, and also offer the options of numerous new beliefs rather than simply focusing on modifying the existing ones.

- Use of prompt cards to summarize points that challenge schemas or reinforce alternative perspectives can be useful. These are utilized as young people will often appear to take on new ideas during therapy sessions but forget them in favor of their traditional beliefs if not reminded. Sometimes, young people will write key prompts that they find particularly helpful on a credit card-sized piece of paper, and get this laminated so they can carry it with them.

- Young et al. (2003) suggested that a key role of therapists is that of "limited reparenting" (p. 182), in which the therapist, within the limits and boundaries of therapy, attempts to provide for the client elements which were necessary but missing from their childhood. Perhaps most obviously, this could involve providing care and support for young people who have grown up in emotionally restrictive or neglectful relationships, but can also involve setting boundaries for young people whose previous relationships have been overly permissive.

- Schema work emphasizes the importance of *emotional* change. Using imagery, role-play, and focusing on historical experiences, schema work relies on evoking strong emotion rather than being an intellectual exercise. Mooney and Padesky (2000) recommended that if a person has difficulties viewing alternative ways of managing a situation, then imagining a role model, or even a fictional character, can be helpful. The case studies later in this chapter illustrate some of these techniques.

- The therapeutic relationship can itself also lead to the emergence of almost any schema, including abandonment, entitlement, enmeshment, approval-seeking, perfectionism, and self-sacrifice. When these become evident, the therapist has a valuable "live" opportunity in which to work. Young et al. (2003) described making the link between a person's schema as it originated from early childhood experience, how it is played out in current relationships, and also how it is enacted in the therapeutic relationship. Davidson (2000) described the interaction between the client and therapist as a "relationship laboratory" (p. 28–30) in which the therapist can observe, in vivo, prevailing patterns which the person enacts, and which also allows the client a safe environment in which to try out new behaviors.

- Helping people identify behavioral patterns that maintain their schema can be important. For example, taking on excessive amounts of work, becoming involved in abusive relationships, or looking after others' needs to the detriment of the young person's own, can maintain schemas and place the young person at risk of relapse. Identifying and helping the young person to change these behaviors can be an important part of schema work. Therapists can work collaboratively with the young person to develop tasks or behavioral experiments (see p. 96) aimed at breaking schema-driven behavioral patterns.

Working with self-sacrifice and unrelenting standards schemas

We have found that a number of young people with bipolar disorder present with "self-sacrifice" schemas. This could increase vulnerability to low mood in response to criticism, or guilt if feeling they have not done enough. Young et al. (2003) suggested that while there may be secondary gain from helping others and being viewed by others as "good," there are also costs if these beliefs are held too rigidly, most notably failure of the young person's own needs being met.

Work on self-sacrifice schemas can include gently challenging the young person's views about the neediness and dependency of others. Analogies such as fitting our own oxygen mask before children's on an airplane can also be valuable. Discussing that failure to have our own needs met may lead to resentment can also be important. Many young people acknowledge disappointment that, on rare occasions where they have asked for help from people they have previously been excessively supportive towards, this has not been reciprocated. Also, similar to unrelenting standards schemas, behavioral experiments, when constructed carefully, can help the young person decatastrophize potential outcomes of not always meeting others' requests. One additional point regarding work with self-sacrifice schemas is that the young person may need to be prepared for negative feedback from others, who may not like the changed dynamic in which the young person no longer does everything they are asked. Case study 5.5 illustrates some of these points.

The second schema we often see with our population is that of "unrelenting standards," where the young person constantly strives to achieve 100% in most, if not all, areas of their life. We believe that this may be associated with bipolar disorder in both the depressive and manic phases. For example, perfectionistic beliefs may drive a person to work excessively hard and expect to manage their disorder without support or medication, with self-care and sleep suffering as a result, and could lead to a manic episode. Conversely, depression may eventuate should the person be unable to meet their own demands, with research indicating that perfectionism may be correlated with increased levels of suicidal ideation (Hamilton & Schweitzer, 2000). Lam et al. (2004) suggested that extreme goal striving, expectations of continuous success, and having to be constantly happy, may lead to self-blame when the person's mood deteriorates, and that the person may become "depressed about being depressed" (p. 198).

When working with unrelenting standards, the use of continuums can be valuable, particularly given that some young people have difficulty with the concept of "good enough" and instead polarize between outcomes either being acceptable or being total failures. Therefore, working with the young person to identify what really "needs" to be perfect can be valuable. Further techniques include identifying the costs and benefits of striving to be perfect, and identifying and exposing the young person to the perceived consequences of imperfection, both cognitively and through the use of behavioral experiments. Specifically, this can involve both estimating the likelihood of the feared event occurring, and identifying the perceived "worst case scenario" if it did. While this can be very anxiety-provoking, when undertaken in "safe" conditions – where the consequences are not significant, and in the context of a strong therapeutic relationship – it can be extremely liberating for the young person. A case study is presented in Chapter 9 that illustrates some of these points.

Case study 5.5: work with self-sacrifice/subjugation schema – Danny

Danny was a 17-year-old student from England who developed bipolar disorder while studying in Australia. He described a long history of feeling it was essential not to let people down and that it was important to be a "nice bloke." He appeared prone to depressive symptoms in the context of feeling responsible when other people were angry or upset, and also of being taken advantage of by other students who would ask to copy his work. At times this would lead to him to having to rewrite all his own work due to fears of being accused of plagiarism, becoming overwhelmed, and experiencing suicidal ideation. Careful assessment and use of the YSQ-L3 (Young & Brown, 2005) identified that Danny endorsed a number of self-sacrifice and subjugation schemas. The therapist believed that this may have contributed to his depressive symptoms, as it appeared that his own needs were rarely met.

THERAPIST: "Danny, we talked a bit last time about how your thoughts or beliefs about things affect how you feel and what you do. Does that ring a bell?"

DANNY: "Yeah. I think we talked about how I just feel that I need to look after everyone all the time. And that sometimes it makes me feel like shit."

THERAPIST: "Uh-huh, that's how I remember it too. I think you also said that you felt like you have been like this 'forever.'"

DANNY: "Yeah, that's it."

THERAPIST (*assessing potential origins of the schema*): "Is there an image in your head of when you first felt like you had to look after people all the time?"

DANNY: "Not really. I've probably always thought it."

THERAPIST (*prompting further, as likely that the belief developed in childhood*): "Sometimes people have memories of particular situations when they remember feeling that belief for the first time."

DANNY: "Um . . . I remember my mum getting sad and annoyed because she felt I never helped her around the house when I was about seven years old. One time she told me I was really selfish."

THERAPIST: "What was that like for you?"

DANNY (*appearing quite tearful*): "Pretty bad. I was just standing there feeling really guilty."

THERAPIST (*assessing whether further incidents contributed to the development of the schema*): "Can you think of any examples when someone gave you praise for putting someone else first?"

DANNY: "Not really . . . (*pause*). Oh, there was one of my school teachers, Mr. Foster, who said he thought I was really smart. And that he thought one of the best things about me was that I was always helping other people."

THERAPIST: "How did it feel when he would say that?"

DANNY: "Pretty good (*pause*). But pretty stressful too."

THERAPIST: "How do you mean?"

DANNY: "Well it was like there was this pressure that I always had to do the right thing. And it also made me feel guilty about times that I haven't thought about people or done the right thing. It feels like quite a lot of responsibility."

THERAPIST: "Is this something that is a problem to you?" (*Assessing whether this schema should be a focus for therapeutic work.*)

DANNY: "Well most of the time it's OK. Sometimes though it means I get really stressed and blame myself if people are not happy . . . Sometimes I even feel like I don't want to keep living if I'm always going to feel this stressed."

THERAPIST: "Can you give me an example of that?"

DANNY: "Yeah, my mum had this birthday party when I was about 14 and I remember being really stressed because there were all these people and I felt it was my responsibility to make sure everyone had a good time. It meant that I wasn't able to relax at all and was just really busy watching everyone and making sure they were OK. It's stupid, but I felt really worried that people, including my mum, didn't have a good time and that it was my fault."

THERAPIST (*summarizing*): "Danny, it sounds like this belief maybe came about through a few important events, including your mum criticizing you for being 'selfish,' but also Mr. Foster praising you for looking after others. But it also sounds like it's pretty stressful for you at times. Can you think of another way of looking at this that would have all the benefits, but not as much cost?"

DANNY: "I could think, 'I'll do my best, and that will have to do.'"

THERAPIST (*sensing that Danny may be placating the therapist and enacting self-sacrifice schemas in the therapeutic relationship*): "Is that realistic for you?"

DANNY (*laughing*): "Not really".

THERAPIST (*sharing the joke*): "Danny, that's a really nice example of you acting out the belief even with us in the session, and trying to make me feel good even if it meant that we don't get to talk about your worries." (*Reflecting Danny's self-sacrifice "live" as it emerged in the therapeutic relationship.*)

DANNY: "I know. Sometimes I don't even know I'm doing it."

THERAPIST: "I guess that's one of the first steps in changing an unhelpful belief. Recognizing when it happens. OK, what would be a more helpful, but *believable* way of looking at it, that we could test out?"

DANNY (*long pause*): "Maybe, 'I should still try to help people, but I'm allowed to say "no" sometimes, and not feel bad.'"

THERAPIST: "Is that more believable?"

DANNY: "Yeah."

THERAPIST: "I was wondering if there are any difficulties with this new belief though?"

DANNY (*pause*): "Maybe that people could be disappointed in me."

THERAPIST (*not challenging that this is a possibility*): "How would you manage it if you felt people were disappointed with you?"

DANNY: "I don't know."

THERAPIST (*identifying a role model*): "You told me before that you are a big fan of David Beckham (English soccer player). How do you think he would manage a situation like that?"

DANNY (*smiling*): "I don't know . . . If he couldn't do something, he'd probably be really nice about it, and say it to them quietly, but in a way they'd listen to."

THERAPIST: "Is that something you think you could try?"

DANNY: "Maybe. Yeah."

THERAPIST (*attempting to anticipate any other difficulties which could jeopardise trying the new schema*): "Can you think of any other problems with trying this new belief?"

DANNY: "It will probably feel weird."

THERAPIST: "How come?"

DANNY: "Well it's how I've always been. It kind of feels normal. And safe. Does that make any sense? Because people don't get angry with me. I think changing it might be hard."

THERAPIST: "You're probably right. Most people keep doing what they're used to even if it doesn't work too well, and it might feel a bit uncomfortable at the start trying to think and do things differently . . . (*pause*) Can I ask something though? What could be good about trying this out?"

DANNY (*pause*): "It could really help me feel free. Take the weight off my shoulders a bit. Not have to do everything for everyone all the time, and to feel OK about it."

THERAPIST (*using double-sided reflection*): "So it sounds like you're saying that if you don't change there is a risk of you continuing to feel stressed and even suicidal at times, and that changing might feel 'weird' at the start, but that the possible gains would be worth it."

DANNY: "Yeah."

THERAPIST: "OK. So, if your new belief is 'I should still try to help people, but am allowed to say "no" sometimes, and not feel bad,' how can we try this out?"

DANNY: "There's this guy, another student in my year, who's asking for my assignment, but I don't want to give it to him this time."

THERAPIST: "What would you normally do?"

DANNY (smiling): "I'd give it to him."

THERAPIST: "And what would happen then?"

DANNY: "I'd feel shit. Like I just gave in."

THERAPIST: "So what's going to be different this time?"

DANNY: "I'm going to politely tell him I can't give it to him."

THERAPIST: "And what will he do?"

DANNY: "He'll probably get angry, or make me feel bad, or both."

THERAPIST: "So how will you manage that?"

DANNY: "I'll try some of the assertiveness techniques we talked about, like not making excuses, not getting off the point, and being a 'broken record.'"

THERAPIST (anticipating that the other student is likely to remain annoyed given that Danny would previously relent): "And if he still isn't happy?"

DANNY: "Too bad."

THERAPIST: "Danny, when you do this, how do you think this will make you feel better?" (Confirming that the behavioral experiment Danny has chosen will be helpful in creating schema change.)

DANNY (pause): "I don't know. I think if I can hold my ground and not get upset or bullied into it, I'll feel pretty good. Because I haven't really been able to do it much before."

THERAPIST: "Are you going to be able to try it, and then we could talk about how it went next time?"

DANNY: "Sounds good."

Role-play and imagery

It can be valuable to undertake role-plays, particularly during the depressed phase, in which the young person is encouraged to take the role of the therapist, while the therapist will state the beliefs typically expressed by the depressed person. In practice, young people often find this extremely challenging initially, and find it difficult to argue against their unhelpful negative beliefs as expressed by the therapist. However, if the therapist can be patient and supportive, this can be a particularly valuable exercise, not only in terms of encouraging the young person to develop challenges to their existing beliefs, but also to allow the therapist to uncover beliefs which the young person may not have expressed previously.

Imagery exercises can also be a powerful means of accessing emotional states and influential schemas (Padesky, 1994; Young et al., 2003). These generally involve asking the person to role-play in as much detail as possible an event in which the targeted schema was activated. The therapist may play the part of a significant other in the scenario, and emphasis is placed on the interaction being in the present tense, rather than historically, as this may be more likely to access important emotional states. The young person is asked to describe what they are thinking and feeling during the exercise, with this allowing the therapist to work on the affect-laden beliefs in the session rather than working with hypothetical examples. It appears that change is more likely to occur if beliefs are worked with when the person is emotionally aroused.

For people who have experienced histories characterized by neglect or criticism, time can be spent during role-plays examining potential explanations of why negative events occurred. For example, a typical assumption made by depressed young people is that their behavior or inherent defectiveness caused the irritability or rejection by a parent, with no alternative explanations having been considered. However, in taking time to examine other explanations, it could emerge that the parent was depressed him/herself, or that critical comments made were in the context of the parent's own difficulties at the time.

Padesky (1994) suggested that these role-plays can also allow for practice of alternative beliefs and behaviors, where, for example, the person can stand up for him/herself against an abusive parent, or ask for the care or support which he/she may have been denied. Typically this can be a highly emotional experience for the young person, should only occur once a strong therapeutic relationship has been established, and should be undertaken near the beginning of a session in order to allow time to debrief.

Behavioral experiments

Behavioral experiments can constitute a vital part of helping challenge and modify unhelpful beliefs, and often require considerable imagination both by the young person and the therapist. As noted in the section on homework and goal setting, involving the young person in constructing these can increase the likelihood of behavioral experiments being attempted. Design of a behavioral experiment involves establishing clear alternative beliefs, testing the validity of these, and establishing exactly what it would mean should various outcomes occur. It is important to be extremely specific when setting up behavioral experiments, as if not constructed carefully, they will allow the young person to maintain their pre-existing unhelpful belief.

Humor and playfulness

The use of humor has been described by a number of researchers and clinicians as a useful therapeutic tool (Blackburn & Davidson, 1995; Wender, 1996), and we find that judicious use of humor can be particularly effective when working with depressed young people.

In a review, Bennett (2003) noted that humor in the therapeutic relationship can be seen as a way of "narrowing interpersonal gaps, communicating caring, and relieving anxiety associated with medical care. Patients also use humour to express frustration with their health and with the medical establishment" (p. 1258).

Interestingly, Levinson et al. (1997) found that the use of humor by primary care physicians – in addition to offering slightly longer appointments, encouraging patients' opinions, and giving information about sessions – led to significantly less likelihood of patients being litigious against their doctor.

A recent paper by Terr et al. (2006) noted the importance of playfulness in therapy with young people, and suggested: "Sometimes we must remind ourselves that play is the natural language of the young" (p. 604). One playful technique which can be useful when working with depressed young people is paradoxical questioning. For example, the therapist could ask: "I'm not sure you're depressed enough. What can we do to make you feel a lot worse about yourself, and make you feel far more depressed?" We find that young people with bipolar disorder will typically be bemused initially, but will then cite examples such as "not see my friends," "stop playing sport," "have lots of time to think about things I've failed at," "drink more alcohol," and "sleep all the time, so I feel guilty about not doing anything." This can be a particularly valuable way for the person to gain insight into unhelpful patterns of behavior or thinking.

Similarly, the use of humor and playfulness can be helpful in illustrating to some young people the unreasonableness of some of their self-critical beliefs, such as in the following case study.

Case study 5.6: Anne

THERAPIST: "OK Anne, can I check this out? You're telling me that you need to be perfect all the time or you're a total failure. Right?"

ANNE: "Right."

THERAPIST: But your friends don't need to be perfect?"

ANNE: "Yeah, that's right."

THERAPIST: "And your sister doesn't?"

ANNE: "Uh-huh."

THERAPIST: "And I don't."

ANNE: "Yup."

THERAPIST: "But you do?"

ANNE (*smiling*): "OK. I get it!"

It appears that the gentle use of humor can assist in developing a positive therapeutic relationship, and can be useful when presenting information, managing difficult situations, and reducing anxiety in the session, both for the clinician and the patient (Granek-Catarivas et al., 2006).

Conclusions

- Research indicates that cognitive behavioral techniques for manic, hypomanic, and depressive symptoms can be an important and effective adjunct to conventional pharmacological treatment.
- The CBT model, incorporating collaborative agenda setting, summarizing, and regular reviews may be a helpful and containing model for young people experiencing depressive, manic, and hypomanic episodes.
- Different phases of recovery require different cognitive behavioral interventions, with acute mania or severe depression tending to require an emphasis on behavioral techniques and managing environmental stimuli, while cognitive strategies, including schema work, may be more valuable later in recovery.
- Initial CBT work can include introducing the cognitive model and helping the person understand connections between their thoughts, emotions, behaviors, and biological factors.
- Constructing a CBT formulation can give the therapist and the young person with bipolar disorder an understanding of relationships between life history, schemas, symptomatology, and relapse risks, and can also clarify foci for intervention.
- Encouragement of mood monitoring can be an important aspect of managing bipolar disorder, but is difficult in young people, who are likely to need assistance with this, at least initially.
- Cognitive techniques include considering alternative explanations to manic or depressive cognitions, utilizing Socratic questioning, managing levels of activity, and undertaking experiments in order to generate more helpful thinking styles.

Social rhythm regulation

There is a time for many words, and there is a time for sleep.

Homer, *The Odyssey* (2007, p. 135)

As discussed in Chapter 1, for many young people, exacerbation of manic or depressive symptoms occurs through a spiral of contributing factors, both biological and psychosocial. Specifically, a young person may have an underlying biological or cognitive vulnerability to bipolar disorder, which results in the reduced effectiveness of the person's "shock absorbers" for significant events. Therefore, when a significant event occurs, he/she may experience more marked cognitive, behavioral, or affective change than would someone without the disorder. Following this, he/she may experience either decreased social or occupational functioning or social withdrawal leading to depression, or increased activity and sleep disruption resulting in mania. These changes may in turn exacerbate the initial mood state, and lead to a cycle towards more marked symptomatology (see Figure 6.1).

Sensitivity to circadian rhythm changes is a key vulnerability factor for people with bipolar disorder (Goodwin & Jamison, 1990). Sleep disruption in particular, which can be caused by substance misuse, medication non-adherence, family tensions (high levels of expressed emotion), loss of regular routines because of long-haul travel (crossing time zones) (Scott, 2003), physical illness, study, or other schedule changes, appears an important trigger for mood disruption. Indeed, Wehr et al. (1987) suggested that reduction in sleep may be the "final common pathway" (p. 201) between the initial occurrence of a life event and the development of manic symptoms. This is supported by evidence that people with bipolar disorder are more vulnerable to developing mania or hypomania after sleep deprivation, with research indicating that up to two-thirds of people with bipolar disorder report social rhythm disruption in the eight weeks prior to a manic episode (Malkoff-Schwartz et al., 1998).

Hlastala and Frank (2006) suggested that sleep disturbance, specifically inadequate sleep, may be particularly common in young people, and offered a number of reasons for this. Firstly, normal adolescent development tends towards a reversed sleep cycle where the young person may want to stay up later than parents or siblings as part of their increasing independence. Secondly, instant messaging allows adolescents to remain in touch with friends late into the night. Finally, adolescents often experience significant variation in their sleep-wake cycle due to staying up late with friends on weekends and sleeping late the following morning, generally followed by having to return to their regular pattern of getting up early again at the start of the week to attend work or school.

Historically, there remains a lack of clarity as to why events that disrupt social rhythm – and specifically those that could be perceived as negative – can lead to mania for some people and depression for others. Understanding this has been a challenge since Freud (1921) observed: "We are without insight into the mechanism of the displacement of a melancholia by a mania" (p. 132). However, the following case study illustrates one possible mechanism for this in a young person with bipolar disorder.

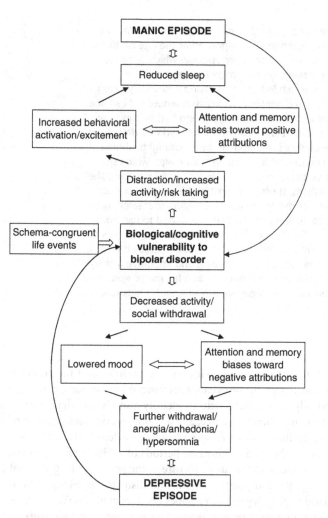

Figure 6.1 A potential model for pathways towards mania or depression for Nadia.

Case study 6.1: cognitive and behavioral mechanisms leading from low mood to a manic episode – Nadia

Nadia was a 22-year-old woman who experienced a number of undiagnosed depressive episodes beginning in her mid-teens. She described that she had always been a "straight A student" but would be vulnerable to experiencing depressive symptoms, particularly guilt, anergia, and anhedonia when she felt she hadn't performed as well as she should have. She stated that since around the age of 16, if she felt she had done badly at school, this would generalize to her recalling and ruminating about a number of other events in her life in which she felt she had performed poorly, and that this would typically lead to her withdrawing socially. Nadia also noted that she would then begin staying in bed and sleeping excessively for weeks at a time "to get away from everything." She described that this would lead to further withdrawal, and that she would then have "more time to think about all the bad stuff." Her academic performance would then suffer, leading to further "evidence" that she was "a retard." This in turn would lead her to further rumination, withdrawal, and hypersomnia. A major depressive episode was diagnosed at the age of 20.

When describing the prodrome to her first manic episode, which occurred at the age of 21, Nadia reported having felt extremely anxious about her performance in upcoming exams, which led to her studying excessively, often late into the night. She had also started drinking an excessive amount of caffeine, through coffee and energy drinks, to assist her studying, and had begun neglecting her self-care. Nadia said that she clearly remembered one day saying to herself: "Screw this." She added that she had then gone out nightclubbing during the week, had attracted considerable attention from males, which she reported had been enjoyable due to her previous poor self-confidence, and she had also started using illicit stimulants, staying up most of the night several times that week. After a number of years of dysthymia and depression, she stated that it had initially "felt great to have some energy" and that she started to feel good about herself, stating that she felt "really popular." Nadia added that she was no longer anxious about speaking to males, and that she wanted to "enjoy it while it lasted." This in turn led her to increased pleasure-seeking and impulsive activity, behavioral activation, and decreased sleep, culminating in a full manic episode.

A diagrammatic model of this was developed with Nadia, and is illustrated in Figure 6.1.

Life event charts

Life event charts may help both the young person with bipolar disorder and the clinician understand the relationship between significant events experienced by the person and the course of their disorder. Specifically, these charts help to identify and visually demonstrate how idiosyncratic life events, stressors, illicit substance, and alcohol use, or medication non-adherence may have contributed to the onset or relapse of manic or depressive episodes.

Importantly, these charts can also be used to illustrate periods of wellbeing and success, which may help provide a more balanced and accurate picture of the person's life, given that state-dependent recall of both negative and positive events and distorted autobiographical memory are common, particularly during depressive episodes (Peeters et al., 2002). It can be especially helpful to include family members or partners in this exercise, while recognizing that some life events, such as sexual history or illicit substance use, may need to be managed sensitively, or discussed later in one-to-one sessions.

In our experience, few young people with bipolar disorder are likely to complete such tasks as homework, and we therefore tend to introduce these as a collaborative exercise during sessions. The young person is asked to add to the chart later should they recall other important events.

Case study 6.2: construction of a life event chart – Brad

Brad was a 22-year-old man who encountered his first manic episode at the age of 18, having previously experienced 2 untreated depressive episodes. Brad described being raised in a country town and that his parents had separated when he was aged 6. While not able to recall the details of his parents' separation, he did remember feeling "sad" at the time. He said that following this he remembered being bullied at school, but that around the age of 11 he started performing well at sports, and became captain of his football team. At age 14 he moved from the country to Melbourne due to his mother finding work in the city. Brad described that he initially found it hard to make friends, and that not long after moving, his grandmother, with whom he was close, had died. Brad added that he began to start playing football in his new school and established some friends and a girlfriend following this. Unfortunately, this relationship did not last, and Brad described experiencing low mood after their break-up, and stated that he began to smoke cannabis at this time.

Brad experienced his first manic episode aged 18, and appeared to make a good recovery, but abruptly ceased taking lithium around 1 year later against medical advice. Following this he experienced a brief period of dysthymia, followed by a second, less severe, manic episode.

The therapist worked with Brad, firstly to identify all the significant events that had occurred in his life, and then to allocate an associated mood rating, between 0 and 10, to each event, plotting these on a timeline (see Figure 6.2).

This allowed Brad to identify some balance in his life history, and to acknowledge some successes and positive events. This was important, given his tendency to self-criticism and preoccupation with perceived failure. It also helped him identify for himself the connection between ceasing lithium and becoming manic, and between his cannabis use and depression, without the clinician needing to take a didactic or overly directive role in emphasizing this.

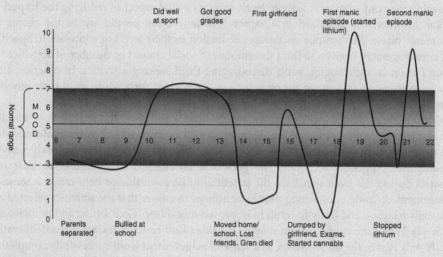

Figure 6.2 Brad's life event chart.

Stabilizing social rhythm

IPSRT was one of the first therapies developed specifically for individuals with bipolar disorder. While there is insufficient space to fully describe the details of IPSRT, excellent overviews of this model are provided in Frank et al. (2000), Power (2005), and Hlastala and Frank (2006). While the model involves assessment, formulation, psychoeducation, and focusing on people's relationships, it also emphasizes the importance of social rhythms. Put simply, Frank et al. (2000) referred to situations, tasks, or people who help us "set our biological clocks" as "social zeitgebers" (p. 595), and that regulation of these can help reduce the likelihood of developing a manic or depressive episode. Therefore, social rhythm therapy focuses on encouraging regular patterns of sleep, eating, exercise, and social interaction, while identifying potential triggers to disruption, and aiming to reduce excessive stress.

While we do not use IPSRT in a structured, systematic way, we feel it is important to be aware of some of the key elements of this model, and that with some modifications it can be useful in work with a young bipolar population. Specifically, we find that the detail involved in completing the social rhythm metric, which involves recording the details of 17 daily activities, makes it unworkable for many young people in the early stages of bipolar disorder. We therefore use a more abbreviated form of monitoring, similar to the adolescent version of the social rhythm metric described by Hlastala and Frank (2006), which we complete collaboratively during sessions, rather than as homework. Typically, this involves inquiring about the young person's daily activities, including the time he/she wakes, starts activity, does sport or exercise, has social contact, and goes to bed. It can also involve recording stresses, daily hassles, mood, and energy levels. While some young people are keen to keep records of this, it is not compulsory and is instead noted by the therapist and reviewed collaboratively during each session. Scott (2001) suggested that even if the individual cannot maintain detailed recording, he/she should be encouraged to establish regular patterns. Eating, going to bed, and getting up can be the most useful activities to target for regularization in the first instance.

Activity levels

Managing the young person's activity levels appears a vital aspect of reducing the impact of bipolar disorder. As discussed in Chapter 5, when young people are in the manic or hypomanic phase the therapist encourages reduction in their levels of stimulation. Specifically, encouragement is given to limit the amount of social contact or number of activities the young person is undertaking, while discouraging thrill-seeking activities. In practice, after a manic episode we encourage young people to "be boring" for a while, until their mood is more settled.

Conversely, as depression is associated with social withdrawal and reduction of activity, a young person in this phase of the disorder should be encouraged to maintain ongoing activity in spite of reduced motivation. This can be managed by using a weekly activity schedule (see Appendix 8), where the person is encouraged to undertake at least two activities during the week that have the potential to be enjoyable or help create a sense of achievement. Socratic questioning should be utilized to ensure that the activities selected are personally relevant, and likely to result in improved mood (see "Goal setting and homework," pp. 80–2). While the young person may be capable of more activities, we often deliberately specify only two in the initial weeks, as a sense of achievement from successfully completing these tasks is more valuable than the risk of failure to reach more ambitious targets.

Sleep disturbance

Decreased sleep is both a symptom of mania and a cause.

Jamison, *An Unquiet Mind: A Memoir of Moods and Madness* (1995, p. 69)

Sleep disturbance can be common in bipolar disorder, with hypersomnia being a characteristic of depression, and insomnia being highly prevalent in depression, mania, and hypomania. When working with young people with bipolar disorder who are experiencing disrupted sleep, it is important to assess all contributing factors for each individual. For example, in addition to biological activation and agitation accompanying hypomania, the clinician should also inquire as to whether the young person is experiencing any cognitive difficulties, including worries, rumination, or excessive planning. Furthermore, it is essential to assess situational and environmental stressors that may be contributing to sleep difficulties, such as noise, heat, brightness, and stress, and the potential impact of medications or illicit substances.

We have found that reversed sleep patterns can also be problematic for a number of young people experiencing bipolar disorder, as they often have an insidious onset and can result in frustration and concern for family members. Typically, if the young person was previously working or studying, this would regulate their sleep-wake routine. However, tiredness during early recovery following a manic episode and commencement of medication often results in stopping study or work, at least temporarily, with this in turn resulting in getting out of bed later in the day. This is likely to lead to a later bedtime, with an altered routine resulting from this.

Sleep hygiene

There is some debate regarding the efficacy of "sleep hygiene" as an intervention, with Harvey (2000) having found that people with insomnia had no poorer sleep hygiene than good sleepers. Similarly, a review by Stepanski and Wyatt (2003) concluded that sleep hygiene interventions, either alone or in combination with other treatments, do not currently have a sufficient evidence base. However, discussing general points which may assist the young person with their sleep can be extremely valuable, and, as Goodwin and Jamison (2007) noted, "there is perhaps nothing more important to the stability of the bipolar patient than good sleep management" (p. 705). Initial work can focus on normalizing tiredness in the early stage of recovery while warning the young person against getting up too late, and encouraging scheduling of activities early in the day to help with getting up at a regular time. We may also advise the following.

Sleep tips

- Avoid napping during the day.
- Avoid stimulants, including caffeine and nicotine (or nicotine patches), especially close to bedtime.
- Avoid alcohol, which although potentially assisting initial sleep onset, can impact negatively on quality of sleep (Stepanski & Wyatt, 2003).
- Try to reduce any noise in the bedroom or outside if possible. Earplugs may help if noise cannot be controlled.
- Have a darkened room in which to sleep, and do not fall asleep with the TV on if possible.
- Try not to have the bedroom too warm or cold.
- Participate in light exercise during the day, but not within two hours of going to sleep.
- Avoid exciting activities close to bedtime (such as some TV shows, playing videogames, or listening to energetic music).
- Have a "wind-down" time prior to bedtime.
- Only use the bed for sleep, not for watching TV, eating, or reading.
- Use relaxation exercises, such as calming music or progressive muscular relaxation.
- If not falling asleep within 20 minutes, get up and do something relaxing. Only go back to bed when feeling tired, and if not asleep within 20 minutes, get up again, and repeat as many times as necessary. Although this may be difficult and tiring for the first few nights, it can help set up a regular sleep pattern.
- It may also be that short-term use of sleep-assisting medication is helpful, particularly if the person is becoming hypomanic. However, this should be a last resort, as evidence suggests that long-term use of some hypnotic medications can result in tolerance and dependence, poorer functioning, increased daytime sedation, and sleep difficulties and anxiety when ceased (reviewed by Riedel et al., 1998).

Sport, physical activity, and diet

Encouraging sport, exercise, and a good diet can be an extremely important aspect of a biopsychosocial intervention for mood disorders, particularly as high rates of weight problems and increased mortality from cardiovascular disease are prevalent in people with bipolar disorder (Angst et al., 2002; Lipkovich et al., 2006). While noting the increased craving for carbohydrates resulting from some medications, Goodwin and Jamison (2007) identified the importance of encouraging the reduction of carbohydrate intake, particularly as "reactive hypoglycemia" can be common in people with bipolar disorder (p. 705). This occurs when the person attempts to combat the negative effects of reduced blood sugar – such as irritability and tiredness that can result from simple carbohydrate intake – by consuming more carbohydrates. Again, if this is addressed early with young people it can prevent the cycle of increasing weight, which can lead to sport or exercise being less enjoyable, resulting in lowered activity levels and further weight gain. However, we recognize that due to increased appetite being common with some medications, weight control can be difficult for many young people.

A second reason for encouraging exercise is due to its positive effect on mood. While a meta-analysis by Lawlor and Hopker (2001) acknowledged that there have been methodological difficulties in much of the research, there is growing evidence that physical exercise can have a significant impact on improving mood for people who are depressed (Babyak et al., 2000; review by Penedo & Dahn, 2005). Similarly, a recent critical review by Ellis et al. (2007) concluded that despite some limitations and lack of consistency in the research, "the findings suggest the presence of a positive effect of exercise on mental health" (p. 95). In bipolar disorder specifically, exercise has been reported to reduce symptoms of stress, anxiety, and depression (Ng et al., 2007).

A third reason to encourage exercise is that it has been found to assist sleep. Goodwin and Jamison (2007) noted: "When at least some exercise is done at approximately the same time every day and not too close to the time for sleep, it can help stabilize circadian rhythms and enhance the integrity of the sleep cycle" (p. 758–9).

When discussing sport and exercise, it appears essential to assist in identifying a pursuit that the young person is likely to enjoy. While this may appear obvious, we have found that young people are highly unlikely to persist with a particular sport or exercise if they do not enjoy it, despite their best intentions. Similarly, consistently participating in regular sport or exercise may be more likely if the young person does it with a friend or as part of a team, as this can aid motivation and social engagement, particularly during early recovery.

Conclusions

- Disruption to circadian rhythms has been associated with the onset of bipolar disorder and risk of relapse.
- For many people, mood can appear to either spiral up or down due to a combination of biological factors, cognitive vulnerability, and behavioral activity.
- Life event charts can provide useful information, but should be undertaken only when the person's mood is stable, with family input being helpful to prevent biased recall relating to current mood.
- Regular patterns of sleep, eating, exercise, and social interaction should be encouraged to help stabilize mood.

Relationship issues and family work

Other things may change us, but we start and end with family.

Anthony Brandt (in Simpson, 1988, no. 3740)

In this chapter we discuss the role of family work in interventions with young people with bipolar disorder. We recognize that family work is a specialized area and highly recommend Miklowitz's (2008) *Bipolar Disorder: A Family-Focused Treatment Approach* (second edition) and Miklowitz and Goldstein's (1997) *Bipolar Disorder: A Family-Focused Treatment Approach*, which have heavily influenced our intervention. We also acknowledge that some of the family therapy literature describes highly detailed interventions, particularly for communication skills and problem-solving (e.g. Mueser & Glynn, 1999). However, as with the rest of this manual, we place a strong emphasis on "real world" work and the following describes interventions that we have found effective when working with our population.

While for simplicity we have included this as a separate chapter, we suggest that in clinical work, the components described and the philosophy outlined should be interwoven throughout the intervention rather than being provided as a discrete module.

The rationale behind family work

There are a number of reasons for including family and relationship work in a psychological intervention for young people in the early phase of bipolar disorder. Firstly, in our population of young people aged between 15 and 25 years, almost 56% were living with their families, or had returned to the care of their families after developing their first episode (Hasty et al., 2006). Therefore, failure to account both for the impact of the family, and for the impact of the disorder on the family, would be to neglect a significant aspect of the person's social environment.

Secondly, family intervention is important given that family variables, including expressed emotion, have a significant impact on recovery in bipolar disorder. Miklowitz et al. (1997) found that criticism, hostility, emotional overinvolvement, or negative, conflictual family interactions led to a considerably higher likelihood of relapse in people with bipolar disorder. Indeed, they suggested that expressed emotion might have a larger effect size on outcome in major affective disorders than in schizophrenia. Similarly, Geller et al. (2002) found that for children with bipolar disorder who were aged between 7 and 16 years, low maternal warmth was correlated with a 4.1-times-higher likelihood of relapse than for those with high maternal warmth. Interestingly, a recent large survey (Morselli & Elgie, 2003) found that people with bipolar disorder reported higher rates of perceived stigmatization in their families than in the workplace (18.1% versus 13.9%). Clearly, therefore, work on psychoeducation for family members and reducing negative interactions is important.

Thirdly, the research on family-focused therapies has generally shown that they are amongst the most useful interventions in reducing symptoms and relapse risk in bipolar disorder (Miklowitz et al., 2007a; 2007b).

Fourthly, it is important to note that family members of people with bipolar disorder are likely to have their own concerns and support needs, may themselves have experienced a mood disorder, or may have difficulties that precede the onset of the disorder in the young person (see review by Goldstein et al., 2002). For example, Hirschfeld et al. (2003) reported that 45% of their bipolar cohort had a family member also diagnosed with the disorder, and Morselli and Elgie (2003) found that 64.8% reported a family history of mental health problems (bipolar disorder in 34.6% of cases, major depression in 43.6%, and anxiety disorders in 15.4%). This is significant, as parental depression has been associated with poorer outcome for adolescents with depressive symptoms (reviewed by Brent et al., 1998). Even for families without any pre-existing mental health difficulties, Miklowitz and Goldstein (1997) urged clinicians not to underestimate the impact of bipolar disorder on the family, and stated that bipolar episodes can represent "a disaster" for the family system (p. 12). While this does not occur for all families, bipolar disorder can pose a significant challenge to parents, siblings, or partners.

Finally, while some of the older literature has been somewhat hostile and blaming towards families, emphasizing genetic loading and expressed emotion, we have found that families can be extremely important treatment allies. Specifically, family members can often assist the clinician during the assessment process, by clarifying the young person's history and premorbid functioning, can help monitor mood and level of risk, can assist in encouraging attendance and medication adherence, and can aid reality-testing and completion of behavioral experiments and homework. Families can also provide an essential support mechanism for the young person, particularly regarding risk of harm, providing practical assistance, and encouraging self-care. It is notable that young people with first-episode psychotic disorders, including a number with psychotic bipolar disorder, have been shown to be significantly less likely to prematurely drop out of treatment when families were included in the treatment process (Graf-Schimmelmann et al., 2006). However, family work is not without its challenges, which will now be described.

Challenges in family work

Similar to individuals with bipolar disorder themselves, family members can hold a number of unhelpful assumptions about the disorder and its management, which can significantly impact on any intervention, whether this is biological or psychosocial. These can include:

- Blaming themselves for the occurrence of the disorder and feeling guilty that some element of their parenting has caused the "breakdown."
- Concern about being "blamed" by others for the disorder, either due to "passing on" the disorder genetically, or by being a "bad parent," due to self-perceptions of neglecting, criticizing, or being overinvolved with the young person.
- Belief that the disorder is purely biological and simply requires medication management, dismissing psychosocial factors or the contribution of family as irrelevant.
- Belief that the disorder is purely psychological or factitious, or that the person simply needs to "get over it" or "grow out of it."
- Feeling guilt due to believing that they should have identified the disorder and sought help earlier.
- Experiencing guilt about the way they responded to the young person during the prodrome. For example, family members may have been critical of the young person's anergia when depressed or their impulsivity when manic, which, in retrospect, they are able to recognize was part of the young person's disorder.

- Difficulty managing the diagnostic uncertainty that may occur in the early stages of service involvement. We find that family members can often be more concerned with obtaining a diagnosis than the young person him/herself.
- Holding a hostile attitude to medication or psychological therapy. This is particularly common if family members themselves have had a negative experience of mental health services, therapy, or pharmacological treatment.
- Underestimating the impact of depressive or residual symptoms, and being intolerant of the young person's inability to function at their premorbid level when experiencing low mood. This may be understandable, as, when depressed, the person may not present as unwell in the same way as they may have done during a manic episode.
- Overinvolvement or overintrusiveness by family members can be common following the first manic or depressive episode, particularly if the person with the disorder is young, has engaged in impulsive behaviors, or presented with suicidality. Family members may also be anxious of relapse, and may become overly intrusive, particularly if feeling guilt for having underestimated or misunderstood prodromal symptoms prior to the first episode. However, overintrusiveness can be particularly challenging in a young, first-episode population where independence issues can be especially important.
- Belief that it is "too late," and that problems have become ingrained. This may result in a sense of hopelessness, or a wish to abandon the young person to be "fixed" by clinicians. This appears particularly relevant if the person has experienced a longer prodrome, or used illicit drugs or alcohol for a lengthy period of time.
- Confusion can exist as to whether behaviors are due to premorbid or emerging personality traits, are normal adolescent behaviors (e.g. wanting to spend more time away from the family, or challenging parental authority), are due to the effects of drugs and alcohol, or are part of the young person's bipolar disorder.
- Confidentiality issues can be particularly challenging when working with a young bipolar population. While older people with the disorder may be more willing for family members to be either involved with, or informed of, their treatment, this is often not the case with young people with the disorder. Specific challenges can include the young person wanting important information to be kept from family members, or family members contacting the clinician without the young person's knowledge and requesting that this is withheld from the young person. It can also include family members exerting pressure on clinicians to disclose details discussed in sessions with the young person. A survey of 1634 teenagers (Gordon & Grant, 1997) identified that many young people reported an unwillingness to speak with a doctor regarding mood difficulties, often due to concerns regarding confidentiality.
- Differing perceptions about bipolar disorder can be a potential source of conflict within families (Miklowitz & Goldstein, 1997), particularly where the young person may under-identify with their disorder and family members overidentify, or vice versa.
- Dissatisfaction or concern should the person be discharged from inpatient care before they are "cured."
- Fear or anxiety by family members about the future, and pessimism regarding likelihood of recovery, can also impact significantly on treatment.

Assessing need

Having highlighted some of the challenges, it is essential that the clinician assesses each family as a unique entity, and designs an intervention accordingly. Similar to engagement in individual work, engaging families should begin with a clear understanding of the expectations, needs, and wants of each member. It is important to note that many families cope extremely well, have excellent communication and problem-solving skills, and do not want "therapy."

Miklowitz and Hooley (1998) noted that bipolar patients and their families appeared irritated by the more didactic elements of a standardized progamme that included psycho-education, communication skills, and problem-solving. Instead, participants appeared to prefer more open discussion about how they had reacted emotionally to issues such as the young person's hospitalization and how symptoms related to the person's premorbid personality. Miklowitz and Hooley concluded that due to the heterogeneity of the bipolar population – including variation in mood cycle length, comorbid substance problems, or Axis II issues – flexibility is required in provision of family interventions for this disorder.

It is also essential to recognize that coping may fluctuate, with members requiring different levels of intervention at different points in time. Generally, in the early stages of contact, more intensive work may be required or wanted by the family. However, as the young person recovers, families typically want less involvement with services, and may only wish to become more involved should there be deterioration or relapse.

Psychological intervention with families of young people with bipolar disorder

Our intervention with families typically involves six components, which are drawn from according to need. These are:
1. Engagement of each family member (including discussion regarding managing confiden-tiality) and "debriefing" around challenging behaviors and difficulty accessing services.
2. Collaborative psychoeducation.
3. Improving communication within the family if this is problematic.
4. Enhancing problem-solving skills.
5. Managing guilt and encouraging appropriate parenting.
6. Mood monitoring and assistance with relapse prevention.

We will address each of these in turn.

Engagement with family members

Engagement often initially involves allowing each family member the opportunity to debrief around issues that may have been traumatic, which can include escalating behavioral problems by the young person prior to contacting services. This can include aggressive or reckless behavior if the young person was manic, or deterioration in self-care, withdrawal, or suicidal behavior if the young person was depressed. Family members also commonly describe frustration regarding having been triaged through a number of different services before obtaining treatment, the time taken to access appropriate help, and annoyance at past misdiagnosis or perceived mismanagement.

The initial phase of family work may also include taking time to inquire about and discuss whether traumatic hospitalization has occurred, including forcible removal, restraint, or police involvement. Allowing the family the opportunity to discuss issues of guilt due to having misinterpreted or underestimated early signs can also be helpful.

It is important for the clinician to be aware that, particularly when working with families of young people after the first episode, members may have little understanding of mental health services. Specifically, families are unlikely to know what they should expect in terms of treatment, and what may be expected of them, and they may need help understanding how services operate. Details of how to contact the treating team, out-of-hours services, and if required, emergency numbers should be provided during the first session.

As part of the engagement process, all family members with whom the young person has regular contact can be invited to the initial assessment session, but may be interviewed separately in the second or third sessions. Including siblings is important, particularly in psychoeducation, as they may have concerns about developing the disorder themselves, particularly if there is a strong family history of mental health problems.

The engagement phase can also facilitate an understanding of family dynamics, of each family member's understanding of the young person's disorder, and how they feel this should be managed. Typically, when working in teams, this can be achieved by one of the clinicians speaking with the young person with bipolar disorder, while another can interview family members separately. Agreement is reached at the end of the separate sessions as to what should be discussed as a group when everyone reconvenes. It should also be made clear to all the participants that the purpose of meeting separately is not to "speak behind people's backs" but to allow everyone to express issues they perceive as important and receive support without fear of distressing other family members or raising unnecessary concern or guilt. The clinicians generally then meet briefly, separate from the family, agree on key points on which to focus, and then give feedback of key issues to all family members with a plan being formulated for management until the next session.

Managing confidentiality

Engagement with families can often require a difficult "balancing act" of meeting the needs of the young person with bipolar disorder and the often differing needs of other family members. Concerns about confidentiality can be a barrier to engagement both for the young person and for their family, and need to be addressed early in therapy. The following are some suggestions that may assist with this:

- The purpose and limits of confidentiality should be explained. It can be important to inform everyone that family members may need to be contacted if risk issues – specifically risk of harm to self or others – are present. However, disclosure of other information to family members should be discussed in the context of the age of the young person, their phase of recovery, and independence issues. While families may find it frustrating that some details may be kept from them, we find that both the young person and their family are generally reasonable around confidentiality issues if clinicians explain their reasons for either disclosing or withholding information.
- We find that it can be important to discuss with the young person that we are keen to involve families wherever possible, and that this is generally something which can be beneficial to the young person. Typically, asking the young person if they feel understood by their family can create open dialogue, as many young people express that they don't feel the family is particularly insightful regarding their experience.
- While we encourage young people to allow open communication about their disorder with their family, we are careful to clarify with the young person which topics are important, how they think their family will respond, and if there are issues they would prefer were not discussed with their family. We find that giving the young person some control over what information is shared with their family usually helps them feel more comfortable about the family being involved in their treatment. If a good therapeutic relationship has been formed, the young person is more likely to trust that the clinician may share information for a good reason, and similarly, families will trust that independence issues may result in some information being withheld.

Taking a "non-blaming" approach is particularly important when engaging families. While this may appear obvious, we find that guilt and self-criticism are particularly prevalent in families of young people with bipolar disorder, at least in part due to initial symptoms often being difficult to detect. Family members often appear to present with an expectation of being criticized by clinicians and may as a result be somewhat defensive. Therefore, addressing blame in the initial session is important.

Collaborative psychoeducation

Individual psychoeducation has been discussed in Chapter 3, and similar principles apply when working with families, namely that it should be provided sensitively and collaboratively. Before commencing any psychoeducation, the clinician should have a clear understanding of each family member's explanatory model, know what they have been told or have read regarding the disorder, and be aware of each member's opinions of the diagnosis and treatment plan. A handout for families, which provides tips on how family members can help the young person with bipolar disorder, is provided in Appendix 2.

As with individual psychoeducation, family psychoeducation should include discussion of what family members have already undertaken to help the young person, what has been difficult, and what has worked well. While this can be challenging if family members have markedly differing understandings of what is occurring, the biopsychosocial model can often incorporate a number of explanatory models (see Chapter 3).

Family work should also include encouragement of hope. "Cautious optimism" should be emphasized, in which it is acknowledged that the young person may be at risk of further episodes, but that there are a number of strategies that can be used to minimize the risk or severity of relapse.

When providing psychoeducation about bipolar disorder it can also be helpful to include discussion of which behaviors are typical of the young person's developmental phase. This may minimize the confusion that families often experience in distinguishing normal adolescent behaviors from symptoms of bipolar disorder. This is particularly applicable when the young person with bipolar disorder is the eldest sibling, and parents have not experienced rebellious behavior or demands for independence with their other children. It should also be recognized, however, that some age-appropriate behaviors may pose risk in terms of precipitating mood symptoms or relapse. Parents may therefore need support in deciding how to respond appropriately to such behaviors, and a problem-solving approach, which is discussed later in this chapter, can be helpful in this regard.

Improving communication skills

Similar to families of people with schizophrenia, communication difficulties are common in families of people with bipolar disorder (Miklowitz et al., 1995). However, people with bipolar disorder have been reported to be more high-functioning, more verbally active, and more likely to defend themselves if criticized, compared to people diagnosed with schizophrenia (Miklowitz et al., 1995; Miklowitz & Hooley, 1998). For example, Miklowitz and Goldstein (1997) reported that, when verbally criticized, people with bipolar disorder are more likely to make comments such as "I don't agree with you" or "I won't do what you're suggesting" (p. 50). This could clearly be problematic and frustrating for families, and may result in an unhelpful bidirectional family dynamic. Put simply, while the likelihood of relapse can be increased by negative expressed emotion, conversely, impulsive, reckless, or irritable behavior by the young person resulting from his/her symptoms is likely to increase the occurrence of further criticism or other negative expressed emotion.

Similarly, amotivation and hypersomnia could lead to negative comments by family members, which may increase the young person's sense of failure and deepen his/her depression.

It is also important to be aware that expressed emotion does not simply comprise negative comments made by family members. Tone of voice and non-verbal behavior such as critical facial expressions or looking away from the person can also be important in discriminating between high and low expressed emotion families (Simoneau et al., 1998). These more subtle types of behavior may be occurring outside the awareness of the family members, and family sessions can be used to identify and carefully address these.

As noted above, expressed emotion has been found to impact on the course of bipolar disorder, and appears strongly related to the beliefs and attributions held by family members about the young person's disorder. Wendel and Miklowitz (1997) found that families who showed high expressed emotion were more likely to believe that the person with bipolar disorder could have more control over their destructive or impulsive behavior if they made more effort. Clearly this has significant implications and should be addressed early by the clinician. Specifically, psychoeducation may help family members understand, and be more sympathetic to, the young person's behaviors that are directly attributable to manic or depressive symptoms, rather than viewing them as willful misbehavior or laziness.

Communication enhancement training

Miklowitz and Goldstein (1997) described "communication enhancement training" which comprises four main skills: "expressing positive feelings," "active listening," "making positive requests for change," and "expressing negative feelings about specific behaviors" (p. 195).

All of these techniques involve making eye contact with the person, being specific about what was liked or disliked about the person's behavior, disclosing what feelings resulted from the person's behavior, and if applicable, discussing how the situation could have been managed differently. Miklowitz and Goldstein also encouraged family members to "catch a person pleasing you" (p. 201), which redirects individuals to a more positive focus.

We find that depersonalizing conflict can also be important. Using expressions such as "when tempers get raised, what is the usual outcome?" or "when people shout, it doesn't seem to help. Could something else work better?" tend to be more effective in assisting behavioral change than targeting unhelpful behavior by a particular individual.

Family communication tips

We advise families and young people with bipolar disorder that a number of techniques can help prevent the escalation of potentially negative situations. These include:

- Choose the timing of raising an issue. If a person is severely depressed or highly irritable, it is unlikely that being critical of their inability to achieve a particular goal or complete a specific task will be helpful.
- Reframe criticism as a request. For example, rather than saying "why don't you help around the house?", this can be reframed as "it's really helpful to me when you do the dishes." The latter comment appears less likely to result in an argument or defensiveness, and targets a specific issue.
- "Pick your battles." Consider how important the issue is before raising it, and if there are numerous issues, decide which are the most significant. Some issues are not worth arguing about at that time, and others may not need to be argued about at all.

- Choose a quiet, private location to have difficult discussions. For example, criticizing a person in front of friends or in a busy shopping centre is unlikely to be effective.
- Use "I" statements. For example, "I'd really like it if you didn't watch me taking my medication all the time. It makes me think you don't trust me" appears more effective than "you really piss me off when you watch me taking my medication. You don't trust me, do you?"
- Keep key points reasonably brief. This is particularly important if the recipient of the message is depressed or elevated.
- Avoid "always" and "never" statements, such as "you never help around the house," "you always watch me take my medicine," or "you're never at home these days." These comments tend to result in the recipient becoming focused on finding examples of when the criticism is not accurate, and are unlikely to motivate the person to change.
- Keep language specific and clear, and do not be distracted onto more general issues. For example, in a situation where the person has spent money carelessly, it is unhelpful to generalize this or be broadly critical, using terms such as "irresponsible" or "selfish." Selecting specific issues may be more likely to lead to a change in the person's behavior than general and vague criticism.
- Avoid shouting, swearing, or other inflammatory language.
- Treat the other person with respect, even when you are being attacked. Keep your tone calm, as it is more difficult to remain angry with someone who doesn't argue back.
- Be aware that how a message is meant, how it is expressed, and how it is heard can be different things. Asking the other person for feedback of how they heard the message can be important. This can be particularly crucial during depressive or manic episodes where interpretations of information can be biased. For example, when depressed, a young person is more likely to perceive a request or advice as criticism, whereas when manic, a person is unlikely to be able to attend to even brief messages.
- Avoid telling the young person that they are behaving in a particular way because they are "sick," "unwell," or "have bipolar disorder." We have found that such labeling can be particularly provocative, and can be seen as pathologizing and belittling of the young person's behavior.
- Take "time out" if required, where family members agree to walk away to another room, or go outside if the situation is becoming emotionally charged. If the situation escalates again, further time-outs may be necessary until everyone is able to discuss the issue calmly.
- Genuinely listen to the other person's point of view, and try to understand why they feel the way they do, rather than using the time when they are speaking to formulate your response.

Therapist modeling can be important in illustrating these techniques, and role-plays can be enacted during sessions, with homework tasks given to practice these between sessions. Role-plays in which the young person with bipolar disorder, the therapist, and family members switch roles can provide a playful way of gaining extremely valuable insights into how family members see each other and therapy.

It can also be very valuable for the therapist to identify "live" examples of challenging issues which occur during sessions, and while being careful not to apportion blame, highlight how a particular comment may have been perceived by the person at whom it was directed. Conversely, it is essential that the therapist is quick to acknowledge strengths within the family, including successful interactions. The therapist should ask the participants why a particular request or comment worked well, so this can generalize outside the therapy sessions.

Finally, it is important that the therapist remembers that families are generally doing the best they can, and that supporting a young person with bipolar disorder can be extremely challenging.

Enhancing problem-solving skills

Problem-solving is described as a significant component of Miklowitz and Goldstein's (1997) family intervention, and involves five steps:

- Identify and agree on the nature of the problem. If there is more than one problem, decide which should be tackled first. Although this may appear simple, it can often be very difficult, and can take considerable time.
- Brainstorm **all** possible solutions, with no possibilities being excluded at this stage, regardless of how unusual or ineffective they may appear. It is important, where possible, to include all family members in this, and to discourage critical comments which may be made in response to some suggestions.
- Discuss the strengths and weaknesses of each option using a grid if necessary, again, with all family members being encouraged to participate.
- Prepare and implement the option(s) that appear to offer the best outcome, devising a plan of when and how the chosen option should be undertaken.
- Assess the outcome and revise if necessary.

Case study 7.1: family problem-solving – Andrew

Andrew was a 19-year-old man who accumulated significant debt when manic. His family was paying off this debt despite having significant financial difficulties, and had considerable concern that Andrew would be at risk of further spending should his symptoms recur.

All family members were asked to "brainstorm" potential solutions, with the therapist writing each of them on a whiteboard. Family members were then asked to identify "pros and cons" of each, until a solution was reached.

PROBLEM	POSSIBLE SOLUTION	PROS	CONS
Andrew spending money recklessly when hypomanic	Take Andrew's credit card away from him immediately	Cease further spending	Will result in Andrew having no money for cigarettes, and appear like we (family) don't trust him
	Ask Andrew what he wants, and buy it for him	Family can monitor what Andrew buys	Andrew loses independence
	Give Andrew allowance in cash	Andrew cannot overspend	Internet items can only be purchased with bank card
	Help Andrew get debit card from bank	Cannot exceed limit	

Agreed solution: set up debit card.

Outcome: Andrew and his mother went to the bank. They set up a debit card with a $300 maximum. Andrew's unemployment benefit payments were sent directly to this account, with a small direct debit organized for board and lodging at home. Andrew expressed being happy about this as it allowed him to spend his own money and retain his independence while removing the risk of accumulating further debt.

Managing guilt and encouraging appropriate parenting

Parents often describe significant guilt about failing to recognize early signs of bipolar disorder. Specifically, parents often express remorse about being overly harsh with the young person due to attributing their impulsivity when manic to deliberate irresponsibility, or attributing the anergia associated with depression to laziness.

As the onset of bipolar disorder often occurs in a developmental context where independence issues are being negotiated, conflict around discipline and rule-setting commonly occurs. When guilt is present, parents may become overly permissive following a manic or depressive episode. This can be unhelpful, particularly if there are other siblings, who may feel resentful regarding the apparently preferential treatment received by their brother or sister. Conversely, parents who feel that ineffectual or absent parenting caused the disorder may attempt to compensate by becoming overly involved in the young person's life.

It appears particularly important to address how parents may have changed their parenting style following the onset of the disorder, and asking the views of siblings can often yield important insights into this. The clinician should help the young person and their family to establish, or re-establish, balance and negotiate appropriate rules, boundaries, and levels of independence.

Mood monitoring and relapse prevention

Ramirez-Basco and Rush (1996) suggested that it can be effective to develop a contract with people with bipolar disorder and their families, describing how each should act should there be indications of relapse. This is best undertaken when the young person's mood is more stable and he/she has some insight into having been symptomatic. The contract can include the young person giving family members permission to contact the treating team if they feel that symptoms are recurring. Having a prepared contract and action plan, preferably written by, or using the wording of, the young person him/herself, can be extremely important. Specifically, this can reduce family members' anxiety about contacting services, and can minimize irritability should the young person start to lose insight during relapse. A case study is described in Chapter 9.

The following is a case study illustrating a number of issues described in this chapter.

Case study 7.2: family work – Corey

Corey was a 23-year-old man with recently diagnosed bipolar disorder. He had lived with friends during the previous year, but returned to live with his parents and younger brother after his inpatient admission. Corey found his parents' increased involvement and direction of his behavior difficult, as he had been largely independent during the previous 12 months.

On first meeting with Corey's family, the therapist inquired about their family history, experience of mental health issues, and understanding of mental health services. Following this, discussion occurred as to how often the family would like to attend appointments, and contact details were provided for the treating team and the after-hours service.

The initial focus of family work involved assessing what the family's experience had been leading up to Corey's contact with services, how his symptoms had emerged, and taking a history as to what may have contributed to him developing bipolar disorder. Corey's parents and brother were also asked how they felt about Corey attending a mental health service and having been admitted to hospital. Close attention was paid to observing interactions between family members in the sessions, noting who was closest with whom, communication styles, and how problems and emotions were managed within the family.

Initial sessions also allowed the therapist to gain an understanding of schemas held by family members, and how these may have impacted on Corey's development and own beliefs. Specifically, his father appeared to hold strong convictions regarding strength and weakness, emphasizing that he himself had never taken time off work due to illness. Conversely, his mother appeared to view Corey's bipolar disorder as inevitable in the context of the world at times being a dangerous and stressful place. Clearly, identifying these beliefs and associated schemas had implications for family work and discussion around psychoeducation. This also highlighted the need to clearly understand Corey's beliefs associated with developing the disorder given the family context.

Considerable time was spent during early sessions gaining an understanding of each family member's explanatory models of what Corey was experiencing. Corey's father appeared to minimize the importance of his symptoms, describing that he felt it was simply "a stage he's going through," and stated that it would not have occurred if Corey hadn't smoked cannabis. In contrast, his mother presented with significant guilt, which was evident when describing an aunt who had bipolar disorder and her concern that Corey may have developed it "from my side of the family." His brother did not offer a clear interpretation as to why he thought Corey had developed the disorder, but noted that their father had always appeared critical of Corey.

Agreement was reached on a psychobiosocial model that attempted to incorporate each of the family members' explanatory models. Discussion of the importance of developmental issues in the onset of bipolar disorder was used to include Corey's father's idea that it was a "stage he's going through," in addition to Corey's substance use, and his mother's conceptualization that he was potentially more vulnerable than others to experiencing symptoms due to stress and genetic factors.

Time was also spent identifying numerous strengths within the family, and on reporting these back at the end of sessions. These included the clear desire expressed by the family to support Corey, their willingness to discuss family dynamics, their interest in education about the disorder, and their attendance at sessions, indicating motivation to assist his recovery. It was also highlighted that family members appeared to complement each other and had supported Corey in different ways. Specifically, his mother was able to encourage his medication adherence and offer emotional support, his father had provided practical assistance and encouraged Corey's self-reliance, and his brother normalized Corey's bipolar disorder by not treating him differently despite awareness of his diagnosis, something which Corey appeared to particularly value.

Issues around independence emerged early in therapy, with Corey becoming irritated that his mother appeared to be watching him extremely closely and that she tended to report to the treating team what he thought were normal variations in his mood. Corey was particularly frustrated that his mother would physically hand him his medication each day and observe him taking it. A session involving Corey and his mother was scheduled to address these issues. While becoming heated and emotional at times, it resulted in Corey having a better understanding that his mother's hypervigilance was related to genuine concern regarding relapse, and also stemmed from her guilt around having not accessed professional help earlier. Corey's mother recognized that her monitoring made Corey feel more anxious and gave the message not only that she did not trust him, but, of even more concern for Corey, that she felt relapse was likely. Corey and his mother used the five-step problem-solving strategy described earlier and decided that he would start managing his medication himself to help him feel more independent. Because his mother was worried that he might forget his medication, Corey agreed to set an alarm on his mobile phone to help him to remember to take it.

When Corey's mood settled, the family assisted in constructing a "relapse checklist" (see Chapter 9), with this including some extremely specific idiosyncratic early signs, many of which were suggested by his brother. While his mother remained somewhat hypervigilant, she became able to reach a more helpful level of concern in the following months.

In later stages of work with Corey and his family, his father admitted with some difficulty that he had initially been somewhat ashamed that his son attended a mental health service, and that he (the father) had been reluctant to attend. Some time was therefore spent discussing his explanatory model of mental health difficulties and stigma issues, and some further psychoeducation regarding the psychobiosocial model of bipolar disorder was provided.

A sense of "cautious optimism" regarding recovery was encouraged, emphasizing the expectation that Corey would continue to get better, but that successful outcome could be assisted by each of the individuals in the room. It was also emphasized that family support, medication, and work on Corey's cognitive style and behavior could reduce the likelihood of his symptoms recurring.

Conclusions

- Many young people with bipolar disorder live with their family of origin, and involving families in treatment can therefore be extremely important.
- Parents and siblings can experience considerable distress, confusion, shame, fear, and a sense of loss early in the course of the disorder.
- Family members can be very valuable allies and can assist with mood monitoring, attendance at appointments, medication adherence, and preventing relapse.
- Discussion with family members regarding their own explanatory models is essential, as this provides the basis for understanding their emotional responses and expectations about recovery.
- Encouraging family members to describe what they have found helpful in assisting the young person when manic or depressed, and acknowledging existing strengths, can be particularly valuable.
- While family work can include psychoeducation, communication skills, problem-solving techniques, guidance regarding appropriate parenting, mood monitoring, and assistance with relapse prevention, this must be done sensitively, collaboratively, and with a clear assessment as to the family's needs.

Alcohol, substance abuse, and other comorbid disorders

When sorrows come, they come not single spies, but in battalions.

Shakespeare, *Hamlet* (1999, p. 701)

When working with many young people with bipolar disorder, managing comorbid disorders – particularly alcohol, substance use, and anxiety disorders – is an integral part of psychological treatment. This is because comorbidity can impact significantly on the effectiveness of other parts of the intervention, including engagement, work with families, psychoeducation, cognitive strategies, social rhythm, the development of sense of self, and relapse prevention. It is also important to note that it may be alcohol or substance use problems that first bring the young person to the attention of mental health services. Therefore, careful assessment can help identify whether the young person may be attempting to "self-medicate" mood difficulties, or whether increased substance or alcohol use is more related to impulsivity or disinhibition.

In clinical practice, work on comorbid difficulties is likely to be integrated throughout the intervention and may not constitute a separate module. The motivational interviewing approach described in this chapter can also be used to assess and enhance motivation to engage in treatment, and to assist with medication adherence. However, as with the preceding chapter on family and relationship work, interventions for comorbid disorders have been included as a separate chapter for ease of reading.

In this chapter, we briefly discuss anxiety and post-traumatic stress disorder (PTSD) in bipolar disorder before focusing in more detail on motivational interviewing approaches to comorbid substance use. We have focused primarily on intervention for substance and alcohol use for two main reasons. Firstly, substance use has a significant impact on outcome in bipolar disorder and is highly prevalent in the youth population. Secondly, interventions for anxiety disorders have been well described elsewhere, with many of the general CBT strategies described in Chapter 5 of this book being applicable in managing these.

Anxiety and bipolar disorder

Careful screening and treatment of anxiety symptoms in young people with bipolar disorder are important as extremely high prevalence rates of anxiety disorders have been found in the bipolar population. For example, a review by Otto et al. (2004) reported rates of panic disorder in 10.6–62.5%, social anxiety in 7.8–47.2%, and obsessive-compulsive disorder in 3.2–35% of people with bipolar disorder. Overall lifetime prevalence of an anxiety disorder was found in 51% of people with bipolar disorder. The overlap between symptoms of mania and anxiety is particularly notable in young people, and a recent study by Biukians et al. (2007) concluded: "Mania and anxiety are not truly independent clinical states in juvenile-onset populations" (p. 75). They also recommended that anxiety in young people with bipolar disorder warrants particular attention due to being connected with higher rates of suicidal behavior.

The high prevalence of comorbid anxiety disorders with bipolar disorder has 3 important clinical implications. Firstly, comorbid anxiety is predictive of poorer outcome in adolescents with depression (Brent et al., 1998), with Conus et al. (2006) finding anxiety was more common than affective symptoms in young people with psychotic mania who did not reach symptomatic recovery at 12 months.

Secondly, we have found that many of our young bipolar cohort appear to experience significantly impaired social and occupational functioning due to comorbid anxiety symptoms, particularly in the early phases of recovery from a manic episode and during periods of depression.

Thirdly, the high rates of anxiety disorders in young people may partially explain the reluctance of this group to engage in treatment, particularly as mania or hypomania may offer a welcome release from the discomfort, social awkwardness, worry, and fear of negative evaluation which can accompany anxiety.

CBT is recognized in the Cochrane database as an effective treatment for anxiety in adolescents (James et al., 2008), with graded exposure being a significant component of this intervention. When introducing graded exposure to young people with bipolar disorder, we find that reverse role-plays can be especially valuable. The following is an example of how this can be done.

Reverse role-play to introduce rationale for graded exposure

We might describe to the young person that we need their help managing our anxiety about water, and that we want to be able to paddle in the sea by next summer, but are currently very fearful of deep water. We would then ask the young person to help or "treat" us for this. While initially bemused, many young people will intuitively describe a graded exposure intervention. If the clinician regularly asks how this will help them conquer their fear of water, young people will often give a very clear rationale behind the process. We suggest that this approach is likely to be more powerful in motivating the young person to attempt graded exposure for their own anxiety difficulties than the clinician describing the process and rationale didactically.

We also find that imaginal exposure can allow for "practice" of a feared situation. This technique involves asking the young person to imagine the situation which they wish to master in as much detail as possible, while encouraging them to "sit tight" through it until their anxiety levels decrease. In practice, asking the young person to close their eyes, utilize all their senses, and describe the situation in as much detail as possible allows for a more realistic experience.

For a detailed guide to cognitive behavioral treatments for anxiety disorders, we recommend Andrews and colleagues' (2003) book, *The Treatment of Anxiety Disorders: Clinician Guides and Patient Treatment Manuals*. This text also provides patient treatment manuals that we find suitable for use with young people with bipolar disorder who are experiencing comorbid anxiety disorders.

Abuse and post-traumatic stress disorder in bipolar disorder

A prospective study by Post et al. (2001) found that people with bipolar disorder who had a history of childhood adversity, including physical or sexual abuse, were more likely to have experienced earlier onset of the disorder, faster cycling of mood, increased suicidality, and more comorbidity with other Axis I and Axis II disorders, including substance use. Post and colleagues also noted that the population who had experienced abuse was more likely to be experiencing ongoing symptoms at two-year follow-up.

A recent review by Leverich and Post (2006) identified that people with bipolar disorder who had childhood trauma had a significantly longer delay before receiving treatment compared to people without an early abuse history (13 years versus 8 years). Their research suggested that this extended delay may partially explain the increased incidence of alcohol and substance use, which may be an attempt to self-medicate.

As in many subgroups of clients who present with mental health difficulties, we recommend screening for evidence of childhood abuse or neglect. Asking about sexual abuse is always a sensitive issue and questions need to be gradually introduced that allow the individual to feel safe in discussing such topics. We recommend screening for sexual abuse specifically by asking questions such as: "Has there ever been a time when someone has touched you in a way that made you feel uncomfortable?" This allows the clinician to ask about abuse experiences in a relatively non-threatening way.

In their review of 1214 people with bipolar disorder, Otto et al. (2004) stated that while estimates have ranged from 7% to 40%, they found a 16% prevalence rate of comorbid PTSD, which they noted was double that of the general population. This has significant clinical implications, with PTSD being correlated with higher rates of substance abuse, increased suicide rates, and lower quality of life in people with bipolar disorder (Simon et al., 2004). However, there is a complex relationship between experiencing traumatic incidents, the development of PTSD, and the emergence of bipolar disorder. There is evidence that while people with bipolar disorder are more likely to have experienced traumatic events, they may also be more likely to experience a traumatic response as a result of their disorder, perhaps most notably involuntary inpatient admissions or police involvement. In addition, a history of trauma puts a person at risk of experiencing further traumatic experiences, impacts negatively on sleep patterns, and may be correlated with lower social support, which in turn may influence the course of PTSD and exacerbate mood symptoms (Otto et al., 2004).

As discussed in Chapter 3, it is also notable that experiencing a mental health problem itself – particularly if this is associated with psychotic symptoms – can be highly traumatic. A review by Gumley and Schwannauer (2006) found that between 11% and 67% of people reported having experienced PTSD following psychosis, either due to symptoms they experienced, or to the associated treatment. While the authors acknowledged that the methodology of a number of the studies was somewhat flawed (e.g. some participants did not clearly meet full DSM-IV [American Psychiatric Association, 1994] criteria), it is unquestionable that police involvement (which may include the use of capsicum spray or restraint) and involuntary hospitalization (which may include physical or chemical restraint) are likely to be traumatic and should be inquired about by the clinician.

Otto et al. (2004) noted that components of CBT which focused on regulating affect and sleep, increasing motivation and self-care, and avoiding substance misuse, may be helpful for people with comorbid PTSD and bipolar disorder. However, they advised that caution may be required regarding use of traditional CBT for PTSD with this population. They suggested specifically that there may be a risk of increased distress associated with exposure to traumatic cognitions or situations as part of the exposure element of treatment. Therefore, they recommended that this can be managed with a strong emphasis on exposure to somatic elements of anxiety during the initial phase of treatment.

Alcohol and illicit substance use

People with bipolar disorder have the highest rates of substance abuse or dependence of any Axis I disorder. Up to 61% of people with bipolar I disorder have a lifetime diagnosis of substance abuse or dependence. Alcohol is the most commonly abused substance (46.2%), and individuals with bipolar disorder are at 5 times the relative risk of alcohol misuse or dependence compared to the general population (Regier et al., 1990).

Comorbid alcohol dependence is important clinically, as it is correlated with poorer medication adherence, increased hospitalizations, poorer outcome in terms of chronicity, and shortened time to relapse in people with bipolar disorder (Keck et al., 1998; Strakowski et al., 1998; Salloum & Thase, 2000). Comorbid alcohol misuse has also been implicated in increased rates of suicide attempts compared to people with bipolar disorder alone (38.4% versus 21.7%) (Potash et al., 2000), and is commonly associated with subsyndromal depressive symptoms (Paykel et al., 2006).

In addition to treatment implications, substance use can also complicate the accurate diagnosis of bipolar disorder, with significant alcohol consumption exacerbating depressive symptoms, and the use of stimulants such as amphetamines leading to elevated mood states. It is therefore essential that clinicians working with young people with bipolar disorder assess substance use, and address this if present.

In addition to alcohol and illicit substance use, cigarette smoking may impact on outcome in bipolar disorder. Smoking was found to double the risk of developing major depression in an epidemiological study of women followed up over 10 years (Pasco et al., 2008). Among people with mental health difficulties, smoking has the potential to worsen clinical outcomes, and reduces the rates of response to acute treatment in bipolar disorder (Berk et al., 2008b). Smoking was also associated with poorer clinical and quality of life outcomes in a 2-year follow-up study of 240 individuals with bipolar disorder (Berk, 2007). It is therefore particularly concerning that smoking rates are disproportionately high in psychiatric cohorts, but this remains a neglected area of integrated care (Olivier et al., 2007).

Engagement and assessment of alcohol and illicit substance use

Young people are often concerned about discussing their substance use with professionals due to fear of legal consequences or disclosure to their family. Therefore it is essential to discuss the scope and limits of confidentiality when engaging and assessing substance use in young people. We find it is also particularly important to explain to the young person that we ask about substance use primarily because of its relationship to mental health and functioning, rather than as a moral or legal issue.

Assessment of substance use can include identifying:
- All the substances the young person has used.
- When the person started use.
- Frequency of use both currently and over the person's lifetime.
- The amount of each substance used.
- Physical or psychological effects when using, withdrawing, or abstinent.
- Use by friends or other family members.
- Patterns of use, including time of day and whether the person uses with other people or alone.
- Under which circumstances the person is most likely to use.
- Risk-taking and impulsive behavior when using or intoxicated (e.g. driving, unsafe sex, or accidents).

- Consequences of use (including family difficulties, effects on physical and mental health, and social, legal, occupational, and financial consequences).
- The longest period of abstinence.
- Whether the person feels able to reduce use if they wanted to.
- Careful interviewing can also identify whether the illicit substance use functions to "self-medicate" emerging mood difficulties, which appears common in this population. Many young people report having commenced cannabis use to manage the agitation or sleep disturbance that may precede a manic or hypomanic episode, or use amphetamines to combat anergia or anhedonia inherent in depression. While use of these substances is clearly not helpful for a number of young people with bipolar disorder, it is important that the clinician understands the person's reasons for use.

Conducting a thorough assessment of substance use with young people and providing feedback of this can be therapeutic in itself (Saunders et al., 1993). Specifically, assessment can assist engagement and facilitate reflection by the young person on their substance use.

Few studies have examined the reliability and validity of screening measures for substance use among people with bipolar disorder, and caution needs to be taken in interpreting their results. Nonetheless, screening tools that may be useful in this population include the following.

The Alcohol Use Disorders Identification Test (AUDIT) (Saunders et al., 1993) is a ten-item measure of harmful or problematic drinking that has well-established reliability and validity in adolescent and adult populations (Allen et al., 1997).

The Alcohol, Smoking and Substance Involvement Screening Test (ASSIST) (World Health Organization, 2002) is an eight-item screening tool for alcohol and substance use which has high levels of internal consistency and test-retest reliability in adult populations.

We find that the Inventory of Drinking Situations (IDS-42) (Annis et al., 1987) can be useful both as an assessment and clinical tool when working with young people with bipolar disorder who are experiencing alcohol problems. This measure is designed to assess the person's perceived likelihood of drinking across eight types of risk situation (unpleasant emotions or frustrations, physical discomfort, pleasant emotions, testing personal control, urges and temptations, conflict with others, social pressure to drink, and pleasant times with others). It can be particularly useful in identifying which cognitive, behavioral, affective, and situational triggers are most likely to lead to alcohol use, which can assist the young person and the therapist in preparing alternative behaviors.

Case study 8.1: use of Inventory of Drinking Situations – Brett

Brett was a 24-year-old man who had been diagnosed with bipolar disorder 10 months earlier, and had begun drinking alcohol heavily during the previous 6 months, after his second inpatient admission. Brett reported that he would drink up to 8 cans of bourbon and cola every day, and that this had led to him becoming more socially withdrawn. He also reported significantly increased tension in the family home, largely due to his increased alcohol use. Brett appeared to recognize that his drinking was problematic and had impacted significantly on a number of goals he had previously held. While appearing keen to reduce his alcohol use, he found it difficult to specify which situations, whether affective, cognitive, or situational, would lead to an increased likelihood of him drinking.

Brett agreed to complete the IDS-42, with Figure 8.1 indicating his responses. Specifically, Brett reported that he was more likely to drink heavily when

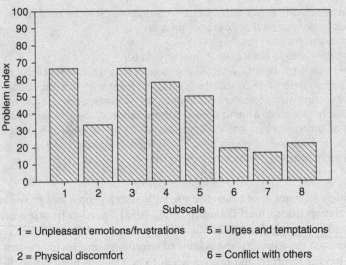

Figure 8.1 Brett's IDS-42.

1 = Unpleasant emotions/frustrations
2 = Physical discomfort
3 = Pleasant emotions
4 = Testing personal control
5 = Urges and temptations
6 = Conflict with others
7 = Social pressure to drink
8 = Pleasant times with others

experiencing unpleasant emotions (such as shame resulting from thoughts of how he had been less successful than his peers), pleasant emotions (particularly, and ironically, to "reward" himself if he had not had alcohol in a couple of weeks), and testing personal control (particularly when feeling confident that he could have "just one drink"). Brett reported finding this exercise particularly helpful as it visually identified high-risk situations, facilitated discussion around his patterns of drinking, and provided the basis for further intervention, which is discussed later in this chapter.

Stages of change and motivation

Prochaska and DiClemente (1986) developed a framework for understanding the stages through which an individual may progress when changing an addictive behavior. This is important clinically as a person's motivation is related to his/her "stage of change" and informs where intervention should begin. These stages comprise:

- **Precontemplation** – where the person may have no apparent insight into their condition and appears unlikely to be considering change.
- **Contemplation** – in which the person may be considering changing the problematic behavior and may be evaluating costs and benefits.
- **Preparation** – refers to the stage in which the person has made the decision to change the behavior but has not yet commenced this.
- **Action** – where the person actually implements changes, such as stopping or reducing their substance use.
- **Maintenance** – in this stage, individuals are sustaining their behavior change.
- **Relapse** – the stages of change model recognizes that relapse can occur. Following relapse, people may re-enter at any of the previous stages.

Young people can vary significantly in their motivation to change alcohol or substance use, and some models for intervening relevant to each of these stages of change are described below. We recognize that there is some debate as to matching intervention strategies to the "stage" in which a person appears to present. Specifically, people may fluctuate in their stages of change even within a session, and there is not a convincing evidence base for stage-matched interventions (William Miller, personal communication, 2008). However, we have found that adapting an intervention to account for the young person's level of motivation can make it more effective.

The following approach has been drawn from specialized texts which we highly recommend, including *Motivational Interviewing: Preparing People for Change* (Miller & Rollnick, 2002), *Cannabis and Psychosis: An Early Psychosis Treatment Manual* (Hinton et al., 2002), and *Self-Help for Alcohol and Other Drug Use and Depression (SHADE)* (Hides et al., unpublished document). However, we would emphasize that the motivational interviewing approach in particular is not simply a collection of techniques, but refers more to a model or style in which to work with people to help them change unhelpful behaviors.

Strategies for young people in the precontemplation stage

In adolescence and early adulthood, autonomy is a prominent issue. Young people generally do not like to be told what to do, and the clinician is unlikely to be effective if overly challenging, or encouraging or expecting change prematurely. This is particularly true for young people who are in the precontemplative stage.

Three general principles of the motivational interviewing approach described by Miller and Rollnick (2002) that can be helpful when working with young people during precontemplation are:

- **Expressing empathy** – using reflective listening demonstrates that the clinician understands the person's opinions and feelings. Care should be taken not to appear judgemental or blaming. Acknowledging to the young person that they are free to make their own decisions creates an environment where the possibility of change can be explored in a non-threatening manner.
- **Unhelpful labeling** – arguing or attempting to persuade the young person to stop problematic substance use is unlikely to be helpful for people in the precontemplative stage, and may result in him/her becoming more defensive or disengaging from services. Ironically, it is also likely to result in the young person voicing arguments *against* change. As Miller and Rollnick (2002) noted, "when you find yourself in the role of arguing for change while your client (patient, student, child) is voicing arguments against it, you're in precisely the wrong role" (p. 22). It is also important to use the young person's own language and avoid use of diagnostic, medicalized, or pejorative terminology such as "addiction" or "alcoholic."
- **"Rolling with resistance" and expecting to be challenged** – It is important to avoid a "clinician knows best" approach or imposing views or goals on a young person. Psycho-education and exploration of harm-reduction strategies can be offered, but it is important to ask the young person's permission prior to giving such information. Encouraging the young person to "take what you want and leave the rest" (Miller & Rollnick, 2002, p. 40), as well as expressing that they have a right to disagree, can result in more open discussion.

Strategies for young people in the contemplation stage

In the contemplation stage, people are typically ambivalent about changing their behavior. Intervention during this phase is therefore aimed at resolving this ambivalence and "tipping the balance" in favour of change. This can be achieved by highlighting the difficulties associated with substance use, while acknowledging the potential benefits of change.

It is important to spend time with the young person to explore and identify the link between their substance use, mood fluctuations, and symptoms or episodes of bipolar disorder. Life event charts, where past and current substance and alcohol use are plotted with the course of the disorder, can assist young people to visually make links between the impact of their substance use and their symptoms (see Chapter 6, p. 101). While psychoeducation can sometimes be useful, it is often not enough to resolve a young person's ambivalence.

Two general principles of motivational interviewing described by Miller and Rollnick (2002) that can be helpful when working with young people who are in the contemplation stage are:

- **Developing discrepancy and eliciting change talk.** This occurs by identifying and clarifying the young person's own goals and values, which may conflict with their substance use. It appears considerably more powerful for the young person to identify these than for the clinician to do so, as goals the clinician might feel are important, such as completing school or good long-term physical health, may not be as important to the young person.

Miller and Rollnick (2002, p. 78–9) suggest a number of open questions that can be useful in encouraging discussion about change, covering areas such as:

- What is the person's biggest concern about their substance or alcohol use?
- How important is it for the person to change?
- What does the person know about the impact of the substance on his/her health even if he/she doesn't feel it is currently a problem for him/her?
- What does the person hope would occur if he/she did reduce or cease substance use?
- How confident is the person, on a scale of 0–10, that he/she could change if he/she wanted to?

When engaging in discussion around change, frequent summaries and reflection can help to reinforce what the young person has said, as well as allow them to elaborate further.

A decisional balance grid can be a useful diagrammatic way to assist with clarifying this ambivalence. This involves asking the young person to write down the costs and benefits of using substances, versus cutting down or not using substances (similar to the medication attitudes matrix in Figure 4.1). While this approach can be helpful with some young people, we advise caution, and are aware of the risks of focusing excessively on benefits of substance use.

- **Supporting self-efficacy.** This involves encouraging the young person to believe that they can change their substance use. Enhancing self-efficacy can be particularly important during depressive episodes where a person may experience hopelessness about their ability to improve or change. If a young person believes they have no hope of changing, they will be less likely to attempt this, despite recognizing the potential benefits of change. Strategies which may assist in enhancing a young person's confidence in their capacity to change can include:
  - Using problem-solving to assist in identifying ways to overcome or manage foreseeable obstacles.
  - Inquiring about existing strengths that the young person can utilize to help them succeed in changing.
  - Reviewing examples of past successes in changing behavior.
  - Reframing past "failures" as "practice," and discussing that most people have several attempts before changing a behavior, and that people often need to try different approaches before they are successful.

Ian was a 19-year-old man with a history of depression and mania. He had experienced a depressive episode approximately 1 year prior to his contact with mental health services, in the context of his girlfriend, Jane, having terminated their relationship. His brief manic episode occurred in the context of substance use and job stress around 6 months later. Ian had not used any illicit drugs during the 4 months following his manic episode, but when the following session took place, he reported having recently recommenced taking ecstasy in the context of nightclubbing with friends.

The therapist was keen to identify not only the difficulties associated with substance use for Ian, but also his reasons for taking it. We recognize that this is a departure from the motivational interviewing literature (Miller, personal communication, 2008), and that it may appear that excessive time is spent discussing benefits of substance use. However, we have found that with some young people, if their idiosyncratic reasons for substance use are not acknowledged (particularly if it appears to have a "self-medicating" role), the therapist may not be viewed as completely understanding the young person's situation, and engagement can be compromised. Therefore, it was felt important to ask open questions and to use summaries and double-sided reflection, in which the therapist would acknowledge both positive and negative aspects of change, so that Ian felt genuinely understood.

THERAPIST: "Ian, one of the things we talked about last time was that you had taken ecstasy and how that was affecting you. Would it be OK if we talked a bit more about that today?"

IAN: "I guess so, but I'm not really that worried about it."

THERAPIST (avoiding risk of confronting or "lecturing"): "OK. How did it go when you took ecstasy last weekend?"

IAN: "It was great. I had an amazing night."

THERAPIST: "Tell me what was good about it?" (Recognizing and prompting for reasons behind substance use.)

IAN: "I just felt really great. Really confident. When I'm doing it (taking ecstasy), it really stops me feeling shit."

THERAPIST: "So what did you do?"

IAN: "I was out on Saturday and Sunday and took pills both nights. My mates and I met some girls. I was so wasted though that I couldn't work on Monday."

THERAPIST: "What happened then?"

IAN (long pause): "I suppose that bit wasn't so great."

THERAPIST: "What do you mean?"

IAN: "Well, it's happened a few times and my boss is getting pretty shitty about it."

THERAPIST: "So you're saying that taking the ecstasy affected you getting to work and your boss is getting pissed off?" (Non-confrontational clarification and reflection of difficulties resulting from ecstasy use.)

IAN: "Yeah."

THERAPIST: "Ian, tell me what's good about ecstasy from your point of view?" (Avoiding risk of only focusing on perceived negative aspects of ecstasy use.)

IAN: "My confidence isn't that great. You know I've been pretty depressed. I've got a real thing about my height and being short and if I don't take a pill before I go out I wouldn't have the confidence to speak to girls."

THERAPIST: "And you feel like the ecstasy helps with that."

IAN: "Sure . . . but I always crash ten times harder."

THERAPIST: "What do you mean?"

IAN: "I feel great when I'm out, but I end up paying for it for the rest of the week. I always seem to feel even worse. And I think a lot about Jane."

THERAPIST: "OK, can I just check back to make sure I'm understanding things properly? You're saying that you are still feeling a bit flat and your confidence isn't always that great. When you take a pill at the weekend you feel good at the time, but it often makes you feel even worse afterwards. It seems to make the depression come back, you end up thinking about your last relationship, and it makes it hard to get to work." (*Therapist using double-sided reflection, identifying both the perceived positives and negatives from Ian's viewpoint.*)

IAN: "Yeah. That's pretty much it. Pretty stupid, eh?"

THERAPIST: "I don't think it sounds stupid at all. In fact it seems to make a lot of sense (*pause*) . . . Ian, I'm wondering a couple of things."

IAN: "Uh-huh?"

THERAPIST: "Well, one is that we could do some work and help you with your confidence and also look at what we can do to improve your mood in the first place. We could also maybe have a think about some things that might help you feel a bit better. To be honest, what we come up with might not be as instantly amazing as the high from ecstasy, but it shouldn't have the costs either, and might help keep your mood a bit more level. What do you think? Would you be willing to give it a go?" (*Acknowledging Ian's reasons for substance use but opening up the possibility of alternative ways of achieving this.*)

IAN: "It's worth a go."

Strategies for young people in the preparation and action stages

The role of the clinician during the preparation stage is to assist the young person to make personal or environmental changes that will help them to change their behavior. As mentioned earlier, many young people with bipolar disorder use substances to "self-medicate" mood symptoms. Where this is the case, exploration of alternative ways to manage acute or subsyndromal symptoms is particularly important.

Anticipating other potential challenges and barriers to change is also important during the preparation stage, including identifying particular situations which could result in increased alcohol or substance use and planning how the person will manage these. Revisiting potential reasons for alcohol or substance use identified in the IDS-42 can be the basis for planning alternative ways of managing these situations.

Because substance or alcohol use often occur in a social context, it can be helpful to encourage the young person to inform their friends that they have an "allergy" to alcohol, cannabis, or amphetamines, and that use could potentially result in relapse or being readmitted to hospital. Preparing the young person for challenging social situations by role-playing clear communication, developing substance refusal techniques, practicing assertiveness, suggesting alternative activities, repetition, or leaving the situation if necessary, can be important. The young person is also reminded that friends who care about them would understand that substance use is not helpful for them, and not push them to drink or take illicit drugs. This can help some young people feel less guilty about assertively refusing their friends. However, we find that many young people who have seen their friends with manic or depressive symptoms tend to be supportive, actively discourage them from substance use, and may even consider reduction or cessation themselves.

Rather than the clinician assuming abstinence is the goal, it is again important to elicit goals from the young person him/herself. The young person may decide to reduce, cease, or use the substance more safely, and the clinician can help create a "menu of strategies," from which the pros and cons of each may be evaluated.

If the young person decides to completely cease alcohol or substance use, it is important that the clinician assists in achieving this safely, such as facilitating admission to an inpatient detox unit. People can also be prepared for withdrawal through information about what symptoms could be expected, and discussion of strategies to cope with symptoms of withdrawal. During periods of acute withdrawal from substances, people with bipolar disorder may need close monitoring for signs of deterioration given withdrawal states can induce mood episodes for some individuals.

It can be useful to create a "change plan" with the young person, similar to that described by Miller and Rollnick (2002, p. 137), addressing the following areas:
- Short-term and long-term goals.
- Main reasons for changing substance use.
- Strategies and steps to help achieve goals (e.g. limits on frequency, quantity, timing, and money spent).
- Strategies to use if feeling tempted to return to old patterns or if experiencing a lapse.
- Possible obstacles or high-risk situations and how to manage them.
- People who can be relied on for help.
- Signs to measure success and rewards.

A change plan is illustrated in the case study later in this chapter.

During the action phase, the clinician can assist with monitoring progress and help revise aspects of the change plan as needed. Advice about potentially successful ways of managing cravings or other temptations may be offered, and activity scheduling (see p. 77) can be helpful in this respect. People may need to be supported through lapses or "slips," with care to ensure that these are not viewed as total failures and therefore a reason to abandon efforts to change. Encouragement of success is also important, with emphasis on ensuring that the young person attributes this to their own actions rather than external forces.

Strategies for young people in the maintenance stage

The final phase in work with some young people with substance use difficulties is that of maintenance, during which the person's changed behavior becomes more established. Maintenance strategies include highlighting successes, encouraging discussion about problems associated with substance use, and identifying positive outcomes that have resulted from the young person changing his/her behavior. It is often important to encourage alternative social, academic, vocational, or sporting activities in order to prevent boredom, and fill the increased time the person may have as a result of ceasing their substance or alcohol use.

Relapse

If relapse occurs, the clinician may use the strategies relating to the phase of change to which the young person has returned. It can also be important to help the young person make sense of the relapse, identify its precipitants, and frame it as a learning opportunity rather than a failure. Problem-solving techniques can be used, and revision of change plans may be needed.

Case study 8.1 (continued): intervention for problematic alcohol use – Brett

As discussed earlier, Brett was able to articulate a number of costs associated with his drinking and already appeared to have some motivation to reduce his alcohol consumption. Although he felt ready to change his behavior, some time was spent eliciting "change talk" to reinforce his commitment to change. This included highlighting the discrepancy between Brett's drinking and his goals of earning more responsibility at work, getting a girlfriend, and saving up money to go on a holiday.

A "vicious cycle" was identified, where Brett acknowledged that his low mood, feeling inadequate compared with his peers, and shame around drinking, led him to consume more alcohol. This in turn resulted in being unable to attend work, withdrawing further, feeling more of a failure, and drinking more. Brett represented this cycle diagrammatically in Figure 8.2.

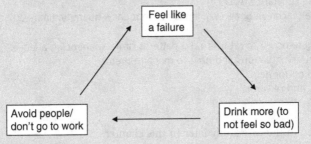

Figure 8.2 Brett's unhelpful cycle.

For Brett, goal setting involved agreeing on a plan where he would try to limit himself to having a maximum of three drinks when with friends, and not drinking at all when alone (a situation which he identified as particularly high-risk). A strategy he thought might help to reduce the number of drinks consumed when with friends was to have soft drinks between every alcoholic drink.

In anticipating potential challenges to change, Brett's clinician described the "abstinence violation effect" (Cummings et al., 1980), with Brett acknowledging that in the past he had viewed any alcohol use as a "total failure," resulting in him feeling overwhelmed with guilt, which had paradoxically led him to drinking more. Specifically, a "slip" (for example a few sips of spirits) had led to him having cognitions such as "I've totally failed. I may as well finish the whole bottle." Attention to this issue focused on discussing with Brett that slips were likely, and that he should prepare for these. It was felt that this would reduce the likelihood of Brett catastrophizing further, and could reinforce the belief that he was in fact still able to cease drinking at any point.

In further preparation, Brett decided to warn his friends beforehand that he was going to reduce his drinking. He told them that he would often become depressed if he drank too much, that he was taking medication, and that if he were driving he would not drink at all. Parts of this had been practiced in role-plays with his clinician beforehand.

With Brett, it was also important for the clinician to acknowledge that one of the major triggers for his alcohol use was low mood. Therefore the clinician was keen to reassure Brett that they would work hard on managing his mood together through psychological interventions and medication.

Brett and his therapist constructed a "change plan," modified from that described by Miller and Rollnick (2002, p. 137), of which Brett had a copy in his own handwriting. It comprised the following:

Short-term and long-term goals
- Get a promotion.
- Get a girlfriend.
- Save some money, and buy a house eventually.
- Go on holiday.
- Get on better with my parents.
- Be more happy.
- Not drink as much.
- Be more healthy, and lose my "beer gut."

Main reasons for cutting down alcohol
- I feel shit most of the time.
- I'm avoiding my mates.
- I've stopped doing anything fun.
- It's costing me money.
- I'm getting fat.

Strategies to help achieve goals
- Put the money I save not drinking in a glass jar so I can see it build up.
- Don't buy as much alcohol.
- Get off the tram one stop before my house so I don't pass the bottle shop.
- Get my mood better so I don't need to drink.
- Only have three drinks with my mates and none on my own.
- Keep busy.
- "Reward" myself in other ways – buy a CD, DVD, or videogame.
- Remember my "vicious cycle."

Strategies to use if craving/feeling tempted to return to old patterns or if I lapse
- Keep busy.
- Go to the gym.
- Talk to myself and remind myself of the bad stuff about when I drink, and how good I'll feel if I don't have a drink.
- "One day at a time" – I just need to make it through the day.

High-risk situations and how I'll manage them
- When feeling shit – call Peter (best friend) or my doctor or case manager. Speak with mum.
- When I've "slipped" and had one drink – remember it doesn't mean anything, and I can still stop if I want to.
- Being given a hard time by mates to drink – do the assertive stuff. "Just say no." Space out alcohol with soft drinks in between.

Supports/people I can draw on for help
- Mum and dad. Probably mum first. Speak with Peter.

Signs to measure success
- See the money build up in my jar.
- Mum and dad happier.
- Feeling better physically (no hangovers and get my abs back).
- Less mood swings.
- Have more energy and feel like seeing my mates.

Finally, it is notable that the motivational interviewing approach and techniques described above can also be used in an integrative way, for example to assess and enhance motivation to engage in treatment, and to assist with medication adherence.

Conclusions

- Young people with bipolar disorder have high rates of comorbid anxiety disorders, excessive alcohol use, and illicit substance abuse.
- Clinicians should assess and manage these sensitively as they are likely to impact on the person's symptomatic recovery, and social and occupational functioning.
- Substance use work can involve assessment, motivational interviewing to enhance commitment to change, setting goals, anticipating challenges, and identifying cues associated with use. There also needs to be a strong emphasis on maintaining change and preventing relapse.

Identifying early warning signs, preventing relapse, and termination of therapy

Prodromal symptoms before manic depressive relapses show considerable variation in their nature and timing between individuals . . . Prodromal symptoms, however, are consistent within individuals giving them a predictive value for each patient.

Perry et al. (1995, p. 405–6)

Research indicates that between 70% and 90% of people with bipolar disorder will have more than one episode (Keller et al., 1993; Gitlin et al., 1995; Tacchi & Scott, 2005), with naturalistic studies showing that around 49.8% of people will relapse within a year, and 68% within 2 years (Silverstone et al., 1998; Lam & Wong, 2005). Amongst those who relapse, two-thirds will have multiple relapses, with 9 being the mean number of episodes (Keller et al., 1993; Gitlin et al., 1995). Given these high rates of relapse in bipolar disorder, work on relapse prevention remains an essential aspect of psychological intervention for this population.

It is encouraging that there often appear to be signs or symptoms which occur before a person becomes symptomatic, with early identification of these providing an opportunity to intervene and prevent relapse. There is also evidence that about 75% of people with bipolar disorder are themselves able to reliably identify their prodromal symptoms for both mania and depression (Jackson et al., 2003), even following a first episode (Ward et al., 2003). In their randomized treatment trial, Perry et al. (1995) found that most of the trial participants had identifiable early signs, which began between two and four weeks prior to a manic or depressive relapse. Two other studies (Molnar et al., 1988; Smith & Tarrier, 1992) indicated that manic prodromes might be longer than depressive prodromes (21 and 29 days versus 11 and 19 days respectively). However, it is notable that people appear better able to identify manic than depressive prodromal symptoms (Scott, 2001; Lam & Wong, 2005), perhaps as the associated behaviors are more overtly abnormal. In contrast, ongoing subclinical depressive symptoms are sometimes misinterpreted as personality characteristics rather than symptoms of an underlying disorder.

A systematic review of 17 studies by Jackson et al. (2003) identified that for mania, sleep disturbance was the most commonly identified prodromal symptom, being reported by 77% of respondents, with psychotic symptoms and changes in mood being the second and third most reported symptoms (described by 47% and 43% of respondents respectively). Mood change, psychomotor symptoms, and increased anxiety were the 3 most commonly reported prodromal signs for depression (48%, 41%, and 36% respectively).

A review by Lam and Wong (2005) noted that the reported prodromal symptoms of depression were more variable, but that common symptoms were "loss of interest in activities or people, not being able to put worries or anxieties aside, interrupted sleep, feeling sad or wanting to cry" (p. 1032).

Egeland et al. (2000) examined prodromal signs reported by family members of children who were later diagnosed with bipolar disorder. Family members reported that changes in mood (53% described depressed symptoms, 38% anger or argumentativeness, and 33%

increased irritability) and energy (47% noted increased energy and 38% decreased) were the most common early signs prior to a first episode.

Identifying personalized early indicators of relapse is important, as this has been shown to improve outcomes in bipolar disorder. A Cochrane review concluded that, while further research is desirable, six high-quality randomized controlled trials indicated that early warning signs interventions were superior to treatment as usual for bipolar disorder (Morriss et al., 2008). The review recommended that early warning signs interventions are "cost effective and worth purchasing" (p. 12) by services, as they increased time to relapse for manic, hypomanic, and depressive episodes, led to a reduction of hospitalization rates, and improved functioning at 18 months.

Psychological interventions for relapse prevention

Taking an individualized approach to identifying prodromes appears particularly important, as, while generalized checklists may not be particularly helpful in predicting relapse, people's idiosyncratic signs appear to have more reliability and specificity. Lam and Wong (2005) summarized this by stating: "Bipolar patients had considerable inter-individual variability but very little intra-individual variability of prodromes" (p. 1032).

Constructing timelines – particularly when the young person has had more than one episode – can be valuable, and can include identifying potential physical, cognitive, affective, environmental, and behavioral triggers which may have led to previous manic or depressive episodes (see Chapter 6 and Figure 6.2). This work can be enhanced with knowledge of the young person's schemas and which specific events are more likely to lead to relapse (see Chapter 5, pp. 70–1). For example, people with "unrelenting standards" schemas may be more likely to experience increased stress and social rhythm dysregulation during times of exams or assignment deadlines. We therefore spend time specifically addressing this and preparing the young person for ways to minimize such disruption, such as ensuring adequate amounts of sleep, creating realistic study timetables, introducing stress management, scheduling breaks and pleasant activities, and cognitive work for unhelpful, performance-related beliefs.

Due to potential lack of insight when relapsing, we encourage young people to have written copies of idiosyncratic symptom checklists. Specifically, we find that it can be useful to complete the three-column relapse checklist described by Ramirez-Basco and Rush (1996) during sessions, with homework for the young person to add further items as they arise. We find this works particularly well when completed collaboratively, and when significant others, such as partners or family members, are included. Typically, this involves asking the young person and family members or friends to describe all the changes they may have noted in the person prior to becoming manic or depressed, including variation in sleep, appetite, interests, thinking, appearance, behavior, activities, and energy levels. Importantly, we encourage people to make this as specific as possible, and have found that the more detailed and individualized this is, the more valuable it can be as a relapse prevention tool. For example, in addition to more general changes, such as with sleep or energy levels, some people report unique variations such as only listening to particular music when becoming depressed, only wearing particular clothes when hypomanic, or wearing considerably more make-up when manic. An example of the detail this can involve is given in Figure 9.1.

Cautions associated with symptom monitoring

While recognizing the importance of constructing early signs lists such as Figure 9.1, we also advise some caution regarding symptom monitoring. While early signs monitoring has been popular in work with psychotic disorders (Tait et al., 2002), a review of prospective

Figure 9.1 Luke's
relapse checklist.

Case study: relapse prevention – Luke

Luke was a 22-year-old man who had experienced 2 significant manic episodes requiring hospitalization. He worked with his therapist to construct the following "relapse checklist," much of which he completed on his own, with additional points being added by family members and from clinical notes.

NORMAL	MANIC	DEPRESSED
Busy, but tired at night	Heaps of energy/not tired	No energy
Good appetite (three meals)	No appetite	No appetite
Some "OK" ideas	New, "brilliant" ideas. Make "connections" between things	Can't think at all
Shy	On top of the world. Really outgoing	At rock bottom
Cry only when something bad has happened	Tearful at times	"Beyond tears"
Sleep around eight hours	Don't feel need to sleep	Sleep all day
Don't write letters and only rarely write e-mails or mobile phone texts	Write heaps of letters/e-mails/texts	Don't write letters/e-mails and don't respond to texts
Feel OK as a person	Feel I'm a movie star and that everything is about me	Feel like "a loser"
Feel I have some control most of the time	Feeling of losing control, a bit like a "runaway train"	Feel no control
Mostly know what's going on	Feel disoriented and confused	Don't care what's going on
Think I'm OK at sport when I train hard	Think I'm brilliant at sport	Think I'm hopeless at sport
Mood around "six out of ten"	"Mood swings" – excited then furious	Mood never above "four out of ten"
Don't worry about my health	Have unusual physical sensations/face feels different	Feel numb physically
Patient with people	Get annoyed if interrupted	Not interested in people
Can stay focused on one thing	Need something to focus on visually	Can't concentrate
Careful with money	Spend heaps of money	Don't leave house
Feel like sex three or four times per week	Feel like sex several times a day	No sex drive
Understand people OK	People's voices don't make sense/sound distorted	Understand people OK
Don't stress about much	Hypersensitive to light/noise	Feel "blank" about everything
Relaxed about being tidy	Need for order	Don't care if tidy or not
Smoke around ten cigarettes per day	Only smoke half a cigarette and then light the next one	Don't smoke at all
Explain things properly	Think people know what I'm talking about and get annoyed when they don't	Don't care if people understand me or not
	Colours look "luminous"	The world looks "dull"
	"Picky" – get annoyed at minor things	Feel like I'm stuck in black mud
	Talk to myself/objects	Very quiet. Serious.
	More suspicious – think people might be jealous of me	More suspicious – think people are criticizing me
	Feel nauseous	Listen to depressing music
	Need for physical comfort/"clingy"	
	Repeat myself	

studies found that it failed to predict between 30% and 50% of relapses (Norman & Malla, 1994). We suggest that if general or vague markers are used, this lack of reliability may be equally likely in bipolar disorder. For example, it is important to note that people should not be encouraged to rely on mood as a marker for potential manic or hypomanic episodes. This is because mood is paradoxically unreliable at the time of relapse, as it is only in retrospect that the individual can recognize that he/she was not "feeling great" but was beginning to become manic (Scott, 2001).

This difficulty may be overcome by assessing the sensitivity and specificity of these early signs. Gumley and Schwannauer (2006) suggested that it is important not only to be able to identify potential signs of relapse, but that these signs should be reliable and responsive to subtle changes. For example, a number of symptoms, including disturbed sleep or increased irritability, while being potential indicators of relapse, are, on their own, often not specific enough to be of assistance to the clinician. Furthermore, hypervigilance for such non-specific signs may in fact create "false positives" in which the person or their family become hypervigilant and unduly alarmed by normal fluctuations in mood or changes in behavior. This may ironically increase the likelihood of relapse. Individual signs can also emerge as understandable consequences of life events, whether positive or negative, and it can be difficult at times to differentiate such normal reactions from prognostically meaningful indicators.

Therefore, discussion should occur with the young person and his/her family as to the reliability of symptoms they have identified as indicative of a potential relapse, as some may tell us little, while others may be clear indicators that relapse is likely. Instead, young people and their families should be encouraged to identify a small number of signs or symptoms which they are likely to remember, and to collaboratively rank these in terms of their reliability. Scott (2001) suggested it is often useful to select one reliable early symptom that occurs at least ten days before a full relapse. At onset of this first symptom, the young person and their family can increase monitoring, with the emergence of a second or third sign in sequence indicating that instituting some form of relapse prevention strategy is required.

Regarding the number of symptoms, with some young men, the concept of a "rev counter" on a car dashboard can be a useful visual tool. This can involve discussion that the presence of three or four symptoms may indicate that the person is in the "mild" range, which may require some action, whereas six or seven symptoms would enter the "red" zone, indicating high risk of relapse.

Relationship between attribution and relapse

In addition to the inclusion of symptom monitoring, we feel it is essential to look at the *meaning* associated with relapse for the person. An emerging literature is evaluating the role of attribution in relapse, and suggests that the meaning a person attaches to early prodromal signs may be highly influential in terms of whether a full relapse eventuates. As Tait et al. (2002) succinctly noted, "if clinicians pay sole attention to the occurrence of specific signs, they risk failing to capture the more holistic and generic meaning experienced by the individual" (p. 143).

In their work with psychotic disorders, Gumley and Schwannauer (2006) described the importance of viewing relapse as an interactional phenomenon, and noted: "Individuals' emotional and behavioral responses to the emergence of early signs of relapse have the potential to accelerate, decelerate or prevent the onset of a full-blown return of psychotic experiences and re-hospitalisation" (p. 33). We believe the same is true for young people with bipolar disorder, as, if a person holds the belief that they are powerless against relapse, this is likely to have a significant impact on their mood, behavior, and, subsequently, likelihood of relapse.

For example, a person may notice that he/she is experiencing reduced motivation. This could be due to tiredness, physical health problems, medication side-effects, or a number of other causes. However, if the person attributes his/her reduced motivation to early signs of a depressive relapse, he/she may feel increasingly anxious and hopeless, and experience a number of negative cognitions. This may affect sleep and subsequent work or school performance, and result in the young person becoming more socially isolated and avoidant of any potentially enjoyable experiences due to fear of failure. Clearly, this could, in turn, lead to a full depressive relapse.

Gumley (personal communication, 2008) also suggested that the clinician's response to potential early signs of relapse can be extremely important, as even subtle behaviors by the therapist may have an impact on the young person. For example, a clinician may generally see a patient alone, but on a particular appointment appear concerned and contact the treating doctor to join the session, or advise an increase in medication. This may communicate that the clinician believes that the young person may be relapsing, and may create anxiety or hopelessness in the young person. While clearly the clinician may have legitimate concerns, and involvement of the doctor may be necessary, we advise clinicians to be mindful of the potential impact of such behaviors.

Beliefs and meaning of relapse

Risk of relapse may be associated with a range of beliefs and responses for young people with bipolar disorder. As discussed in Chapter 3, following a first episode it is not uncommon for young people to deny having bipolar disorder and reject the likelihood of symptom recurrence. Alternatively, some individuals believe that becoming hypomanic would be a positive experience, and that they would be able to keep it under control without becoming "unwell." Undertaking relapse prevention work without addressing these beliefs is likely to be met with resistance or derision.

Tait et al. (2002), in their early signs monitoring work, described the importance of discussing with people what thoughts and memories are associated with previous episodes or are related to thoughts of relapse. They also reported asking people to describe which associated events were the most distressing, what the events meant to the person, how the person saw themselves in relation to the disorder, and what cognitions, affect, and physiological signs were associated. For example, some people report feeling powerless, guilty, ashamed, angry, or embarrassed, with this leading to a marked fear of relapse. Gumley and Schwannauer (2006) noted that a number of these emotions may be experienced simultaneously by the person, with, for example, the image of being alone in a psychiatric hospital involving associated emotions of humiliation, anxiety, and sadness.

Therefore, we find that it is important to comprehensively assess the young person's cognitions and beliefs relating to relapse. A tool which can be helpful to assist with this is the Attitude to Relapse Scale (Appendix 11: Davies, unpublished), which specifically assesses fear, catastrophization, and perceived control over relapse. Sentence completion tasks can also provide the clinician with a good understanding of the young person's cognitions regarding relapse. This can include asking the young person to finish sentences including:

- If I relapse, then . . .
- If I lose control . . .

- If I get stressed . . .
- If I start feeling depressed . . .
- I can prevent a relapse by . . .

When people present with maladaptive beliefs about relapse, a cognitive approach can be utilized. This can include evaluating the accuracy, costs, and benefits associated with these beliefs, how the person would like things to be, and finding evidence to support more helpful alternative beliefs. Clinicians may need to spend some time decatastrophizing the perceived impact of a relapse, particularly if the young person associates recurrence of symptoms with beliefs of permanent disability, social rejection, isolation, or inability to function.

Managing a potential relapse

Relapse prevention work can include asking the young person how they plan to cope themselves and how they would like to be managed by others should they re-experience depressive or manic symptoms. On occasion it can be helpful to have a written copy of this, but time should be spent realistically discussing who should be in charge of the checklist and plan, and what input from others the young person would accept. The purpose of the exercise is identification of a collaborative management strategy, rather than something that the young person feels could be used by family members or the treating team as a means of control.

Typically, this involves identifying possible "first," "middle," and "late" signs of a potential depressive or manic relapse, and clarifying how the young person, family or friends, and the treating team should respond (see Appendix 12). While many young people are initially only able to identify more extreme symptoms, this can nonetheless be a valuable exercise if constructed collaboratively over several sessions.

Card-sort activity for relapse prevention

A card-sort activity can serve as a useful prompt to help young people identify early signs. While Lam et al. (1999) recommended that people with bipolar disorder should be guided to provide descriptions of their early warning signs using their own words and without prompts, Agius and colleagues (2006) noted that many people have difficulty providing detail about prodromal signs without specific cues. Therefore, they encouraged the use of a card-sort activity after first asking the patient to describe what happened prior to the first episode or relapses.

Common prodromal experiences identified in the literature (e.g. Smith & Tarrier, 1992; Agius et al., 2006) can be listed on a piece of paper, following which the young person selects items that occurred during his/her prodrome. The items identified by the young person are then discussed so that general signs can be made more specific (e.g. "increased creativity" may be more specifically elaborated as "stay up late drawing and painting"). Idiosyncratic signs that are not represented on the list can also be added at this point. Cards are then made of each of the items and the young person is asked to arrange these in an approximate order, from the first thing he/she noticed through to the last thing that occurred. These can then be grouped into categories of: "first signs", "middle signs," and "late signs." A more personalized approach involves making cards of each of the early symptoms identified by the young person and his/her family from the three-column relapse checklist (see Figure 9.1) and asking the young person to arrange these in order of progression.

Relapse prevention plans typically include both cognitive behavioral techniques (described in Chapter 5) and interventions designed to stabilize social rhythms (described in Chapter 6).

WHAT TO LOOK FOR	WHAT TO DO	
FIRST SIGNS	MYSELF	FAMILY/ FRIENDS
Feeling more excited and confident. Being more talkative. Having heaps of energy.	Remember that mood changes could be because of normal everyday things. Ask dad and Gillian (my girlfriend) if they think anything's going on (mum gets too stressed and thinks *everything* is a relapse). Make sure I'm not getting to stressed or doing too much. Make sure I'm taking my meds. Make sure I have an appointment in the next few days. Make sure I'm getting enough sleep (about eight hours). Cut down on cola and coffee. Not too much coffee, and NO ENERGY DRINKS!	Not to panic (or get tearful or angry). Not to tell me I'm "relapsing." To check with me that I've got another appointment. Gently check that I'm taking my meds every day (even though I hate being asked).
MIDDLE SIGNS	MYSELF	FAMILY/ FRIENDS
Getting annoyed and snappy more often. Feeling a bit more suspicious. Making more "connections." Thinking things on TV or people talking might be about me. Half-smoke cigarettes.	Slow things down and "be boring" for a while. Read more. Party less. Listen to R&B instead of dance music. Listen to the doc, and increase my meds if advised to.	For my parents or mates to ask if it's OK to call my case manager or doctor. Make sure that I'm sleeping and eating OK.
LATE SIGNS	MYSELF	FAMILY/ FRIENDS
Not sleeping at all. Thinking I'm a movie star. Being sure that people are watching me. Talking all the time. Thinking too fast.	STAY CALM! Try to listen to my parents and remember they are not trying to upset me. Take sleeping tablets if advised to, even though I feel like staying up.	STAY CALM! Take me to see my doctor and case manager (even if I think I don't need to). Take me to hospital (if I **REALLY** need to).

Figure 9.2 Relapse prevention plan for potential manic episode – Luke.

Figures 9.2 and 9.3 are examples of relapse prevention plans. They were both completed by Luke, whose case is described in Figure 9.1. The first is his plan for a potential manic relapse (Figure 9.2), and the second for a potential depressive relapse (Figure 9.3).

WHAT TO LOOK FOR	WHAT TO DO	
FIRST SIGNS	MYSELF	FAMILY/FRIENDS
Sleeping a bit more and not feeling like getting up. Being more "serious." Making excuses and not going to the gym.	Make sure I'm still keeping active. Don't panic!	Encourage me to keep doing stuff, even if I say I can't be bothered (but not too much!) Don't automatically think I've stopped my meds.
MIDDLE SIGNS	MYSELF	FAMILY/FRIENDS
Missing days at school. Not feeling like eating as much. Feeling a bit flat and not seeing my friends as much.	Phone for an extra appointment even if I can't be bothered. Try really hard to keep doing things. Remember I've felt like this before but I've always got myself out of it.	Get in touch with my case manager or doctor if I haven't already done it.
LATE SIGNS	MYSELF	FAMILY/FRIENDS
Don't feel like doing anything. Feel hopeless. Feel like I'm wading through black mud. Avoid everything.	Go to appointment or let mum, dad, or Gillian take me in. Remember I've got over this before.	Take me in to hospital if really needed, but only as a last resort.

Figure 9.3 Relapse prevention plan for potential depressive episode – Luke.

Schema work in preventing relapse

As mentioned in Chapter 5, there has been research indicating a correlation between particular schemas and vulnerability to relapse in bipolar disorder (e.g. Ball et al., 2003; Lam et al., 2004). Therefore, as part of relapse prevention, working with young people to modify schemas that may put them at risk of relapse appears important.

Case study 9.1: schema work to prevent relapse – Jasmine

Jasmine was an 18-year-old woman who developed a manic episode following intermittent periods of depression. She made a good recovery from her manic symptoms after commencing a mood stabilizer. She presented as very likeable, articulate, and insightful, but clearly found it difficult to describe her previous depressive symptoms, instead tending to divert the sessions towards more superficial subjects which she felt more comfortable discussing.

Jasmine completed the YSQ-L3 (Young & Brown, 2005), but reported afterwards that it had been quite emotionally challenging for her. While her scores remained low for most of the subtests, indicating that she did not strongly hold potentially unhelpful beliefs for these domains, her scores on two subscales were highly elevated. Specifically, on the self-sacrifice subscale, she indicated that the statements "I'm only happy when those around me are happy" described her perfectly, and the statements "I put others' needs before my own, or else I feel guilty" and "no matter how much I give, it is never enough" were mostly true of her. On the unrelenting standards subscale, she strongly endorsed "I often sacrifice pleasure and happiness to meet my own standards" and "almost nothing I do is quite good enough; I can always do better."

It was discussed with Jasmine at the outset that therapy was not going to attempt to fundamentally change her beliefs, as, generally, these were highly adaptive, and clearly contributed to her academic success, popularity, and aptitude in her part-time job. However, Jasmine was insightful that her perfectionism, and poor attention to meeting her own needs, could put her at risk of relapse.

It was noted during family work that Jasmine's parents, particularly her mother, held very similar beliefs about success and the importance of putting others' needs first. Jasmine identified that her own critical self-talk about "not trying hard enough" was reminiscent of comments made by her mother to her when she was younger. Jasmine was encouraged to judge the accuracy and helpfulness of these critical comments, rather than accepting them as fact.

It was not long before Jasmine's schemas would have an impact on her mood. She attended her tenth session, and initially presented as confident and euthymic, briefly stating that she was feeling good, and then diverting the session towards the therapist's wellbeing. With gentle use of humor, the therapist identified that Jasmine was something of an expert at taking care of others, even her therapist, but that this often appeared to result in Jasmine not having her own needs met or addressing her own difficulties. At this point, Jasmine became tearful and reported that she had experienced a fairly difficult week. Specifically, she stated that she had been accused by her father of being "selfish" regarding a financial incident. The therapist discussed that it was understandable that this was especially upsetting for Jasmine given her self-sacrifice schemas and the importance for her of putting others' needs first. Further discussion confirmed that criticism relating to this would be one of Jasmine's "hot buttons" which would be likely to elicit a strong emotional response, specifically feeling angry and ashamed. It had also led to increased rumination and sleep difficulties for her. It appeared important to rationalize with Jasmine why this event, although possibly innocuous to others, was important to her, as she tended to be highly self-critical regarding perceived oversensitivity.

Jasmine then reported a second incident, describing having competed in a sport in which her mother had previously been a coach. Jasmine had only recently taken up the sport, but came second in a local competition. As could be expected, Jasmine stated that she felt this was not good enough, and believed she had disappointed her mother by not coming first. The therapist asked Jasmine what would have happened if she had won, and what would have been her mother's response, to which Jasmine responded: "She probably still wouldn't have been happy, because she didn't think the girl who won was that good." This question, and further Socratic interviewing, appeared to clarify for Jasmine that her mother's standards could often be unreachable. Discussion also identified that Jasmine often appeared to put herself in situations which were "unwinnable," and where even success could be negatively reframed as "not good enough."

Following this, work with Jasmine focused on helping her identify situations in which her schemas were unhelpful, encouraging her to be slightly kinder to herself, and to recognize that meeting her own needs as well as those of others were not mutually exclusive. It was also important to work with Jasmine to identify which demands or expectations by others were excessive, and how she could manage her guilt in refusing unreasonable requests. Specifically, in response to Jasmine's father's comment about her being selfish, Jasmine was encouraged to take a "mini time-out" when feeling upset in the future, in order to assess the fairness and accuracy of the other person's comments. She acknowledged that she had previously been unable to do this, and instead tended to accept and become preoccupied with any criticism, no matter how unreasonable.

Initially Jasmine felt it was too challenging to discuss her parents' criticisms with them directly, so the "empty chair" technique was used so that she could practice voicing these issues to her absent parents during a session. While she initially felt awkward doing this, it quickly became a fairly emotional experience for Jasmine, with her becoming tearful. At this time, Jasmine also disclosed a critical incident that clarified a possible contributor to the etiology of her unhelpful schemas. Jasmine reported that as a ten-year-old she had been asked to watch her five-year-old sister Gillian as they swam in a local pool. Gillian had momentarily gone under the water for which Jasmine had been strongly criticized by her mother, who told her: "If either of you were to die, I would prefer if it was you." Clearly this had a significant impact on Jasmine, who later acknowledged that she felt she had been "defined" by this incident. The importance of this was discussed in terms of Jasmine's schema formation, with Jasmine being able, towards the end of therapy, to recognize that her mother's response was extremely hurtful and unfair. Jasmine was also able to identify that the comment had been made when her mother was angry and frightened, and also occurred in the context of Jasmine's mother having been shown little affection by her own mother. Exploring this appeared important for Jasmine who had previously – due to extreme shame about the incident – taken her mother's comment as evidence of Jasmine being a selfish and unlovable person.

While Jasmine initially found it difficult for the therapist to see her upset, schema work appeared to be important in four main respects. Firstly, it allowed Jasmine to verbalize some of the difficult emotions she had been experiencing, which she had not previously disclosed due to extreme shame and guilt, in addition to not allowing herself to be "pathetic." Secondly, it appeared to challenge her underlying belief that she was worthless if not taking care of others. Thirdly, therapy allowed Jasmine to consider how she might like to raise some painful issues with her parents. Finally, it provided her with a clearer indication of which events were likely to lead to her experiencing low mood, and informed her of ways to attempt prevention of these through cognitive and behavioral means.

Relapse prevention plans

Case study 9.2: prevention of a depressive relapse – Simone

Simone was a 25-year-old woman who had experienced untreated mild to moderate depression for a number of years prior to presenting with a manic episode.

Similar to Luke, described earlier in this chapter, Simone completed a three-column checklist, and identified a negative cycle she could get into when depressed,

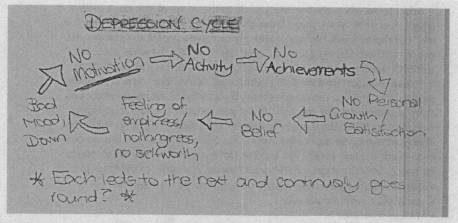

Figure 9.4 Simone's negative cycle. Reproduced with many thanks to S. M.

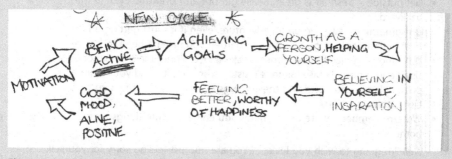

Figure 9.5 Simone's positive cycle. Reproduced with many thanks to S. M.

drawing a diagram of this (Figure 9.4). She also recognized a positive cycle of behavioral techniques she could utilize to help improve her mood (Figure 9.5).

When she was in the recovery phase, Simone was asked to write a letter to her "depressed" self, giving advice on what she could expect and how to change negative patterns. This proved particularly valuable, as Simone composed a compassionate and reassuring letter to herself, describing her unhelpful beliefs and schemas. She specifically identified absolute demands she placed on herself that she "must" or "had to" achieve particular goals. It also helped her anticipate her own destructive thinking and behavioral patterns, including hopelessness about recovery, in addition to describing practical and personalized coping strategies, which had worked for her previously.

Simone's letter to herself

Dear Simone, hello my old friend. We've been through some tough times together, especially lately . . . I know at times you just can't see the point of everything or anything but guess what? There doesn't have to be a point, or even better find out for yourself what the point is, 'cause I know if anyone else tries to tell you what the point is you won't believe them anyway. You see I know what it feels like where you are, I know how bad it can be. But I also know how much better it can get . . .

Now I know when you feel like you do at the moment you don't believe in advice. You think "yeah, yeah I know that sounds good but it won't work for me," but I know it will, I've seen it with my own eyes, I've felt it. Knowing you, you are still skeptical so I'll do you a deal. Just try it. What have we got to lose? Just STOP for a moment. STOP and we'll take a break. Let's have a holiday from ourselves, just for a week to start off with. Remember you don't **have** to do anything, and you can do everything if you want to. Along the way if you think of something else you want to do, you can, there are no rules except one – just try. If you do, that's an achievement in itself. There is no failure, no disappointment; you are not letting anyone down. In fact, if you like, no-one even needs to know except you and me. I love you and all I want is for you to be happy. So let's escape – here's your itinerary, try some of the following:

- Be nice to yourself – have a bath, do something with your hair . . .
- Make your environment nice . . .
- Talk to someone.
- Challenge your thoughts – try to find both sides to each one and let's just go with the happier thought for a while.
- Get outside – fresh air is great. Really get out and **breathe**. Even in the backyard.
- Do something new – go on an adventure, even if it's just getting on the train with a book, or go to a park or garden you haven't been to before.
- Do something nice for someone – make a nice dinner for Billy (Simone's boyfriend) or buy Louise (Simone's sister) a small gift, send your mum a poem. I know you like doing these things even if you don't feel up to it.
- Listen to music/sing.
- Write/remember – write down things you enjoyed, write things that bothered you.

Well I'm going to wish you luck . . . You are not just feeling sorry for yourself, you are not abnormal, mental or a freak. You just walked off the path a little and I'm showing you the way back. So if you are thinking "fuck this," well fuck you because I'm never going away. Believe me I know we are meant to be together, as we are the same person, we are Simone.

(Reproduced with many thanks to S.M.)

Simone also constructed a plan when at risk of a potential depressive relapse, which consisted of:

- Attending increased outpatient appointments (two per week).
- Work looking at negative cognitions (particularly self-criticism).
- Reading the letter she had written to herself.
- Increasing activity levels, including maintaining her gym attendance and scheduling positive activities (seeing her sister and going to the cinema), while recognizing this would initially be difficult for her.
- Recognizing "crap excuses," a phrase which Simone used to describe reasons she would automatically generate to avoid a situation which she found challenging. These included "I'll do it tomorrow," "it's too cold/hot today," "I'll do it next week when I feel better," "I don't have any money," "I'd need to get two trains to get there," "I don't feel like doing it today," "there's something on TV I really want to watch," "if I can't do it as well as I used to do, there's no point in doing it at all." Simone had written these on a list that she stuck to her bedroom mirror, and was even able to display some humor when she became aware of using them.

- Attempting to reduce her amount of sleep to nine hours per night, and setting a regular time to get out of bed. This was important, as hypersomnia had previously resulted in increased self-criticism, guilt, and further anergia and hopelessness.
- Liaising with her employer, with whom she had a good relationship, to support her in her workplace.

Time was also spent with Simone discussing the meaning of relapse. She acknowledged that she had initially considered relapse as inevitable, a personal failure, and as further evidence that she was "weak." The therapist worked with Simone on the strength of her conviction relating to these unhelpful cognitions. At the end of therapy, while she retained some concern both about likelihood of relapse and her responsibility for this, the degree of conviction and the associated distress were significantly reduced.

Termination of therapy

The progress a patient makes during therapy should be enriched and heightened by a positive treatment ending. When termination issues are ignored or mishandled, the whole of therapy is jeopardized.

Kramer (1990, p. xv)

Good planning and preparation for termination of therapy can be extremely important when working with young people with bipolar disorder. The therapist may have played a significant role in the young person's life, and it is likely that the young person could experience some sadness or anxiety regarding their future without the therapist. Ryle and Kerr (2002) noted: "As termination is approached, the absence of anxiety and disappointment would suggest that the reality of the end is not yet felt by the patient" (p. 113).

When working with young people who have had difficult attachment histories – particularly those with associated abandonment schemas – clinician sensitivity and allowing time to discuss issues around finishing work together are essential components of therapy. The cognitive analytic therapy literature suggests that termination should be on the agenda from the first session, as this allows both the patient and clinician to plan for the end of therapy, and emphasizes the importance of utilizing all sessions fully (Ryle & Kerr, 2002). While discussion of this at the onset of therapy may not be appropriate when working with someone who is acutely manic or significantly depressed, it can nevertheless be important for the therapist to be aware of termination and to raise it early in the course of therapy.

Kramer (1990) suggested: "To each patient, termination means something different" (p. 63), and therefore, different types of endings – such as reducing the frequency of sessions, taking "breaks" when the person is asymptomatic, and having an "open door" policy once therapy has officially ended – may all be appropriate depending on the patient. While specifics of termination may be at least partly defined by service considerations, we find that even at the successful conclusion of therapy, many young people and their families retain some anxiety regarding the possibility of relapse. Therefore, it is not uncommon to receive phone calls or occasional visits from young people who have officially finished with the service. We feel it is important to be available, whenever possible, in these situations, even if the main focus is on ensuring that the young person has another service with which to engage.

It is also important for the clinician to have time to acknowledge his/her own thoughts and feelings regarding the end of therapy with each patient. While workplace demands may mean that there are constantly other patients waiting, we suggest that time to reflect on termination, and if possible, not having another appointment immediately after a final session, may be helpful. As Kottler (2003) noted of finishing therapy, "the clinician may feel guilt, failure, disappointment, sadness, pride, apprehension, hope, jealousy and relief – all at once. And there is the constant cycle of growing immensely fond of people and then turning them loose" (p. 94).

The goodbye letter

Termination of therapy can be an emotional experience, both for the clinician and the young person, and is an opportunity to reflect on successes of work together, and on goals that have not yet been achieved. Utilizing a technique described in the narrative therapy and cognitive analytic therapy literature, we have found that a "goodbye letter" can be a valuable therapeutic tool. While we recognize that there is not currently an evidence base for utilizing this technique with a young bipolar population, we find that a letter allows for reflection around key issues that have emerged during therapy, describes the joint understanding reached regarding the disorder, and is also a record of the therapy for the young person to keep. We would stress again that similar to the CBT formulation letter described in Chapter 5 (p. 73–6), prior to writing the goodbye letter, collaborative discussion should occur as to what it should include. If necessary, both parties can take notes in final sessions, with the degree of involvement by the young person in this being largely determined by their developmental level. The therapist can then provide the young person a typed version incorporating all that was discussed.

The goodbye letter

Typically, the letter would include:
- Identifying some of the key issues that the person presented with during therapy.
- Briefly outlining the shared formulation. This includes making the link between the person's history, development of schemas, and how symptoms may have related to this, and summarizing the collaborative biopsychosocial model of the person's experience.
- Describing the progress the person has made, and their plans and goals for the future. If psychometric measures such as mood questionnaires or graded activity schedules were used, reference to these can also be valuable.
- Reporting on agreed plans on how to minimize likelihood of relapse and giving a message of "cautious optimism."
- Importantly, it also allows for the therapist to reflect on and, where appropriate, disclose their own experience of therapy with the young person. This can include describing what challenges they have experienced, what they have appreciated about the young person, and what the clinician him/herself has learned from the experience.

It can be valuable to not only give the young person the letter, but also to read it to them during one of the final sessions. This can allow for discussion around what the therapist may have missed, and can also be an opportunity for the therapist to receive feedback about key messages the young person has retained, what the person has not found particularly helpful, and what was valuable about the therapy. Discussion at this point can allow for a final opportunity to correct any misunderstandings, and also for the therapist to model that sadness, disappointment, and anxiety, in addition to hope, may be appropriate. While recognizing that there may be numerous ways in which a goodbye letter can be written, the following is an example that includes some of the key aspects described above.

Case study 9.3: goodbye letter – Natalie

Dear Natalie,

As I promised, I wanted to write you a letter summarizing some of the things that I think have been important during our work together. It will also be good to hear your thoughts about this too.

When we first caught up, you seemed pretty angry at "having to go to a psycho hospital," and I think a lot of the things I said at the start really annoyed you. I'd guess that it was pretty frustrating that you were sure that there was nothing wrong, and everyone else was saying something different. However, you managed to keep coming to see me, and after a few weeks, you began to tell me some really important things about your life and how you thought about things.

You told me that it was pretty tough growing up in a house where your dad was depressed, and that you felt you had taken on some of your dad's "issues" without even meaning to. For example, you told me that, like your dad, you could sometimes be a fairly pessimistic person, but that it was "safer" to be that way, because then you would never be disappointed. You also told me that, whenever you would start feeling happy, you would pull back, and it was like having your dad's voice in your head telling you to "settle down" and "pull your head in."

You explained to me that there were some advantages about thinking the way you did, and that it could be "protective" for you. But you also said that it would make you worry a bit too much sometimes, and that you could never "allow" yourself to enjoy things as much as your friends seemed to, and that, sometimes, you would be "scared of being happy." You added that at times you could be pretty down on yourself and wouldn't feel like doing much.

Even though these beliefs were there before, I wonder if having a manic episode confirmed them even more, because, when you did allow yourself to be happy, it got a bit out of control and you ended up in hospital.

We have spent a bit of time talking about the good things and bad things about how you used to think, with you saying that you thought it would be good to be a bit happier, and that you wanted to be able to "think a bit more positively." As we discussed, sometimes in the past it seemed that being critical of yourself and other people was a really good motivator. You said it allowed you to achieve a number of goals, while making people "back off." But you also told me that when it hasn't worked, it has really sucked, and has been very destructive for you.

Even though it was quite hard when your mood was a bit flat, you were able to give me examples of things that you could do each week that would make you feel even a little bit better. You would then try them out and tell me how they went, like when you started going back to the gym.

We have also spent a lot of time figuring out new thoughts that would be more helpful, but still believable. You worked on your "new language" of less negative thoughts, which was really hard at the start, but you told me recently that you think you are getting much better at it. Like we discussed, it will take ongoing work to keep some of the old critical thoughts in check, and the old thoughts are probably still the first ones to pop into your head. It seems though that you are now able to think about "what else could be going on?", rather than just accepting the old thoughts as facts.

I wonder if one of the most important things for you to keep working on after we finish is to be a bit more gentle with yourself, but I think you are well on the way to being able to feel more happy. Getting the right amount of sleep (not too much and not too little!), regular contact with your friends, going to the gym, and going to school, even when you didn't feel like it, has also seemed really important in helping keep your mood OK. I wonder if the medication has also helped, but I know you're not sure about that.

Finally, we spent some time looking at how to prevent any of the depressive or manic symptoms coming back. While this seemed difficult at the start because you probably weren't that keen to think about it (which is pretty understandable), you were able to write a pretty good list of really reliable signs to be aware of. You also have a pretty good plan of what to do if anything does come back. We also spent some time talking about what it would mean if any of the symptoms do come back, and figuring out ways not to freak out about it.

I have been really impressed with how hard you have worked during our time together, even though it might have been weird and difficult to do things differently. I also wanted to say that I have really enjoyed our sessions together. I have especially appreciated your sharp wit, our conversations about psychology, and the fact we have been able to work together even though you have not always agreed with me. You have also given me some great examples that I will be able to use with other people, like saying your energy level was like a car battery and that the more you did, the more energy you'd have.

It has been great working with you.

Best wishes, and I'm confident that if you keep up your hard work, you'll continue to go really well.

Yours sincerely,

Conclusions

- Relapse prevention work appears essential given the high rates of symptom recurrence in bipolar disorder.
- While some heterogeneity has been identified in terms of prodromal symptoms for manic and depressive episodes, it appears important to obtain a unique "relapse checklist" for each person.
- Timelines can be used to help identify potential physical, cognitive, affective, and behavioral triggers that may have led to manic or depressive episodes.
- Symptom monitoring work should aim to identify a small number of highly specific, memorable markers, and how many, how intense, or for what duration symptoms need to have lasted to constitute a relapse. Paradoxically, mood does not appear to be a helpful marker, particularly in terms of manic relapses.
- While symptom monitoring can be helpful, it can also create increased anxiety and hypervigilance. Clinicians should therefore work with young people and their families to achieve a balance between awareness of potential early signs, while discouraging unhelpful hypervigilance.
- Time should be spent with the young person and their family identifying attributions and the meaning associated with relapse, while decatastrophizing beliefs about symptom recurrence.
- A "relapse plan" can be constructed, including how the young person would like to manage emerging symptoms themselves, and what input they would want and would accept from family and professionals.
- Termination of therapy can be challenging for both the young person with bipolar disorder and their clinician. However, if adequately planned, it can be an extremely valuable opportunity to summarize and highlight key points of therapy, in addition to providing encouragement about the person's own self-efficacy and ability to effectively manage their disorder.

A checklist of the key interventions described in this manual is provided in Appendix 13.

Appendix 1: A guide for people with bipolar disorder

What is bipolar disorder?

Bipolar disorder, also known as manic depression, affects at least 1 or 2 in every 100 people.

Bipolar disorder is a mood disorder involving extreme changes in emotion. While anyone can experience "ups and downs," bipolar disorder can result in a person at times feeling extremely happy, excitable, and invincible, and at other times feeling irritable, miserable, or even suicidal. Bipolar disorder can also affect the way people think and behave, can affect work, study, and relationships, and can result in hospitalization. It is also a disorder that can keep returning if not treated properly. However, it can also be managed very effectively, with evidence showing that getting help earlier can result in better outcomes.

Diagnosis should only be made by a health professional, but symptoms can include the following:

Symptoms of mania

Feeling "high," full of energy, or easily annoyed **for at least 7 days, and:**

- Feeling "driven" to do things, which may feel out of control at times.
- Reckless or impulsive behavior and doing things you usually wouldn't, e.g. spending excessively, being more promiscuous, making decisions without thinking them through, or using drugs or alcohol excessively.
- Finding it very hard to concentrate or focus on one task, and not being able to finish tasks.
- Feeling physically jumpy.
- Talking very fast.
- Feeling like your thoughts are going very fast, or jumping from one subject to another.
- Feeling like you don't need any sleep.
- Increased sexual drive.
- Increased self-confidence.
- Feeling you have special abilities or talents that no-one else has.

Symptoms of depression

Feeling sad most of the day, nearly every day, or not enjoying activities you did before **for at least two weeks, and:**

- Feeling hopeless.
- Feeling slowed down, with it being hard to have the energy to do things you would previously have found easy.
- Feeling guilty without a reason.
- No longer enjoying things you did before.

- Problems concentrating.
- Sleeping much more, or finding it very hard to sleep.
- Eating much more, or not feeling like eating.
- Thinking about death or suicide.

Sometimes people can experience a "mixed" episode, where there are symptoms of both mania and depression at the same time. This is particularly common in young people.

People can also experience some psychotic symptoms when they have bipolar disorder, involving a loss of contact with reality, which can include hallucinations or delusions.

It is important to remember that while anyone can experience these symptoms, with bipolar disorder, a person would experience a number of them at the same time or for long periods of time.

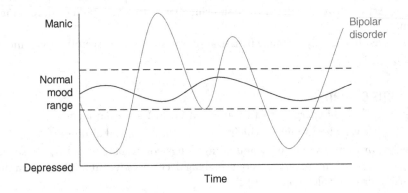

What causes bipolar disorder?

There does not seem to be one single cause for bipolar disorder. A number of explanations have been suggested as causing bipolar disorder, including genetics, brain chemistry, and stress.

Genetics – people have a greater risk of experiencing a mood disorder if a first-degree relative (brothers, sisters, or parents) has experienced one. If a person has 2 bipolar parents, or an identical twin with bipolar disorder, he or she will have a 60–65% risk of developing it.

Brain structure and chemistry – researchers have found some differences in the brains of people with bipolar disorder including enlarged ventricles and changes in the release of neurotransmitters like serotonin, norepinephrine, and dopamine.

Psychological factors – stress appears to play a major role in the development of bipolar disorder. People often first develop bipolar disorder in their late teens and early twenties, which can often be a time of significant life events, like exams, moving out of home, finding work, and developing important relationships. It also seems that a lot of stress in families can lead to more relapses, and some recent evidence suggests that particular personality types may be more vulnerable to developing bipolar disorder.

In summary, people seem to develop bipolar disorder through a combination of factors including stress, the way they think about things, and biological vulnerability.

How do we treat bipolar disorder?
Medication

- People diagnosed with bipolar disorder can be prescribed different types of medication. The most common is a **mood stabilizer**, such as lithium or sodium valproate. Mood stabilizers are not addictive, and work by balancing the brain chemicals which may be involved with depression or mania. If people are also experiencing hallucinations or delusions, they may also be prescribed an **antipsychotic** medication such as olanzapine, quetiapine, or risperidone.

- Mood stabilizers can take two to three weeks to work, and work best when they are taken consistently. They are used for treating people when they are in the acute phase of the disorder, but can also be very important in preventing mania or depression from returning.

- Mood stabilizers require monitoring and blood tests, and it is important to take them at the prescribed dose, and to only reduce or stop them under medical supervision.

Therapy or counseling

Psychological treatments have been found to help prevent extreme mood swings, reduce hospitalizations, and improve people's functioning. They often involve providing information about bipolar disorder and its treatment, looking at reasons why the person may have developed the disorder, identifying possible triggers which could cause relapse, and looking at the thoughts and behavior that can keep the person well.

They can also involve looking at structuring, and finding balance, to activities in the day, including encouraging the person not to do too much when they are manic, or too little when they are depressed.

Counseling or therapy can also involve the whole family, particularly if the person is still living at home. This can be helpful in reducing stress, and in working out helpful ways to talk to a person when they are manic or depressed.

What can I do about bipolar disorder?

- Get help early, as this can prevent the disruption and distress that bipolar disorder can cause, including relationship difficulties, family stress, and financial, employment, and study difficulties.

- Seek help from a health professional such as a doctor or case manager.

- Keep taking your prescribed medication and don't be tempted to stop it when you feel better without discussing it with your doctor or case manager first.

- Avoid making any important decisions (e.g. changing jobs/study courses, spending large amounts of money, moving home, starting new sexual relationships, getting tattoos or piercings etc.) when either manic or depressed.

- Illegal drugs (such as cannabis or amphetamines) or excessive alcohol or caffeine can make symptoms worse or cause relapse. Try to limit use of these, or not use if possible.

- Seek a balance between doing too much activity and too little.

- Pay attention to sleep patterns, as too little sleep appears to be a major factor in triggering and maintaining manic episodes, and too much sleep can be related to depression.

- Find time to relax and do some light exercise.

- Learn to identify your own symptoms and personal triggers.
- Try to trust and listen to people who care about you, as you may not recognize when symptoms are coming back.
- Avoid risky behavior (gambling, extreme sports/driving fast).
- Listen to, or read stories from, other people who have bipolar disorder.
- **Remember that this is a treatable disorder.**

For further information, please contact your doctor/case manager. (Also see additional handout in Appendix 2: "What can I do to help a person with bipolar disorder? – A handout for family members and friends.")

Appendix 2: What can I do to help a person with bipolar disorder? – A handout for family members and friends

- Encourage the person to attend appointments, recognizing they may need your help to do this either due to lacking energy when depressed or being disorganized when manic.
- Encourage the person to take their medication, but be aware that this may be a sensitive area, and may require negotiation and discussion.
- Discourage drug or alcohol use, while recognizing that the person may be using these in an attempt to deal with their symptoms.
- Encourage the young person to reduce stimulation, including too much activity, late nights, loud music, or too much excitement when he/she is manic or at risk or becoming manic, while being aware that he/she may become frustrated or angry with you for intervening.
- Encourage the person to try to keep a regular routine of when they sleep, eat, and exercise. Again, this can be difficult when the person is acutely unwell, but is worth focusing on when the person is more settled.
- Help the person do more activity when depressed, while recognizing this may be very difficult for them.
- Try to remain patient, as the person's inactivity when depressed or impulsive behavior when manic is unlikely to be due to laziness or deliberately being difficult.
- Keep calm and speak gently to the person when they are either depressed or manic. Shouting or becoming annoyed is unlikely to help the person change their behavior and may make things worse.
- Try to behave as normally as possible. Simply ignoring the person or being overly involved with them may not help.
- Gently discourage the person from making impulsive decisions. Encourage them to delay major decisions until their mood is settled, or to seek the advice of someone else if your opinion is not enough for them.
- Have a good idea of what the person's symptoms are when unwell and know what warning signs to look for should they relapse, but remember that some "ups and downs" can be normal depending on what is going on for the person.
- Have a "relapse drill" or plan of what to do should the person become unwell. Ideally, this can be planned out and agreed upon by everyone.
- Have contact details of the person's case manager, doctor, or crisis team handy and don't be afraid to contact them if you are concerned.
- Know how to look after yourself and make sure there is someone you can talk to about your own worries or concerns, as caring for someone with bipolar disorder can be extremely stressful.

Appendix 3: The bucket metaphor

What factors do you think might have contributed to you developing your bipolar symptoms? (For example, family history, substance use, school/work stress, relationship issues, family difficulties, high standards, other life experiences, etc.) "Fill" the water level of the bucket giving the appropriate amount for each factor. Please also identify factors which "drill a hole" in the bottom of the bucket, or increase the size of your bucket to stop it overflowing (e.g. taking medication, stress management, family support, seeing friends, not using drugs, or other things which help you cope).

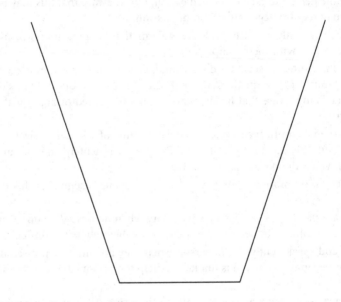

Appendix 4: Repertory grids

Good	1	2	3	4	5	6	7	Bad
Reliable	1	2	3	4	5	6	7	Not Reliable
Popular	1	2	3	4	5	6	7	Alone
Confident	1	2	3	4	5	6	7	Shy
Smart	1	2	3	4	5	6	7	Stupid
Stable	1	2	3	4	5	6	7	Unstable
Predictable	1	2	3	4	5	6	7	Unpredictable
Free	1	2	3	4	5	6	7	Trapped
Healthy	1	2	3	4	5	6	7	Sick
Accepted	1	2	3	4	5	6	7	Isolated
Rational	1	2	3	4	5	6	7	Irrational
Independent	1	2	3	4	5	6	7	Dependent
Calm	1	2	3	4	5	6	7	Irritable
Understood	1	2	3	4	5	6	7	Misunderstood
Happy	1	2	3	4	5	6	7	Sad
Hopeful	1	2	3	4	5	6	7	Hopeless
Creative	1	2	3	4	5	6	7	Boring

(Please note that other categories can be added which may be personally relevant.)

Appendix 5: Views on bipolar disorder questionnaire – Hayward et al. (2002)

In this questionnaire, the person is asked to indicate on a six-point Likert scale ranging from "strongly agree" to "strongly disagree."

	Strongly agree			Strongly disagree		
1. Most people would willingly accept a person with bipolar disorder as a close friend.	1	2	3	4	5	6
2. Most people believe that a person who has been hospitalized with bipolar disorder is just as intelligent as the average person.	1	2	3	4	5	6
3. Even though I have experienced bipolar disorder, I feel just as capable as the next person of getting and holding a job.	1	2	3	4	5	6
4. Most people believe that a person with bipolar disorder is just as trustworthy as the average citizen.	1	2	3	4	5	6
5. Most people believe that entering a psychiatric hospital is a sign of personal failure.	1	2	3	4	5	6
6. I am able to do things as well as most other people.	1	2	3	4	5	6
7. Most employers will inform a person who has experienced bipolar disorder if they are qualified for the job.	1	2	3	4	5	6
8. Even though I have experienced bipolar disorder it has not affected my ability to sustain close relationships.	1	2	3	4	5	6
9. Most people in the community would treat someone who had experienced bipolar disorder just as they would treat anyone.	1	2	3	4	5	6
10. Most young people would be reluctant to date a person who had been hospitalized for bipolar disorder.	1	2	3	4	5	6
11. Once they know a person has been in a psychiatric hospital, most people will take their opinions less seriously.	1	2	3	4	5	6
12. There have been many occasions when I have avoided social situations because of my bipolar disorder.	1	2	3	4	5	6
13. Having bipolar disorder makes it more difficult for me to make friends.	1	2	3	4	5	6
14. I feel I am a person of worth, at least on an equal plane with others.	1	2	3	4	5	6

Reproduced and modified with very kind permission of Peter Hayward.

Appendix 6: Medication attitudes matrix

ADVANTAGES OF TAKING MEDICATION	ADVANTAGES OF NOT TAKING MEDICATION
DISADVANTAGES OF TAKING MEDICATION	**DISADVANTAGES OF NOT TAKING MEDICATION**

Appendix 7: Blank CBT formulation

The clinician and young person with bipolar disorder work together to complete the following CBT formulation.

Early history

Core schemas

Conditional beliefs

Critical incidents   Affective/cognitive impact

Maintaining factors

Cognitions (auto thoughts)   **Affect**   Behavior

Protective factors

(modified from Fennell, 1989, p. 178)

Appendix 8: Weekly activity schedule

This can be completed either before undertaking activities or on their completion.

Day/time	Mon	Tue	Wed	Thu	Fri	Sat	Sun
7–10 am							
10–11 am							
11–12 am							
12–1 pm							
1–2 pm							
2–3 pm							
3–4 pm							
4–5 pm							
5–6 pm							
6–7 pm							
7–8 pm							
8–9 pm							
9–12 pm							
12–7 am							

Appendix 9: Mood monitoring chart

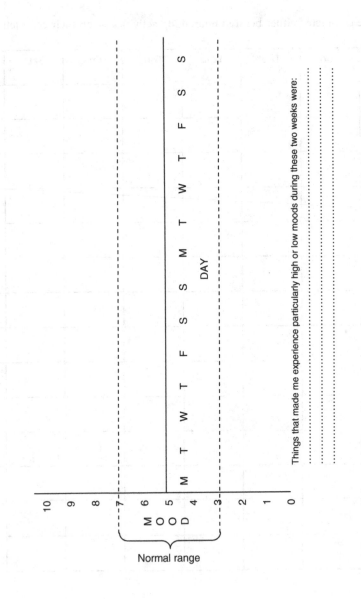

Things that made me experience particularly high or low moods during these two weeks were:

Appendix 10: Responsibility pie

INTIAL BELIEF(S)	STRENGTH OF BELIEF	ASSOCIATED AFFECT

Cognitive therapy work

Identify what other factors/other people may have contributed to the outcome. Brainstorm all possibilities no matter how minor they may be, and allocate the percentage influence they may have had.

Responsibility pie

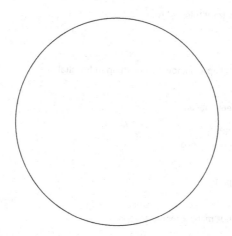

REVISED BELIEF	STRENGTH OF BELIEF	ASSOCIATED AFFECT

Appendix 11: Attitude to relapse – Davies (unpublished)

Reproduced with kind permission of Ellen Davies-Edwards.

A. Fear

I worry about relapse every day

| Strongly agree | 1 | 2 | 3 | 4 | 5 | strongly disagree |

The possibility of relapse is something I have learned to live with

| Strongly agree | 1 | 2 | 3 | 4 | 5 | strongly disagree |

I rarely worry about relapse

| Strongly agree | 1 | 2 | 3 | 4 | 5 | strongly disagree |

Although I try not to, I often find myself worrying about relapse

| Strongly agree | 1 | 2 | 3 | 4 | 5 | strongly disagree |

The possibility of relapse is something I'll never get used to

| Strongly agree | 1 | 2 | 3 | 4 | 5 | strongly disagree |

B. Catastrophization

If I begin to show signs of relapse, I know I will end up in hospital

| Strongly agree | 1 | 2 | 3 | 4 | 5 | strongly disagree |

If I begin to relapse I will feel a failure

| Strongly agree | 1 | 2 | 3 | 4 | 5 | strongly disagree |

If I begin to relapse, I will not go mad

| Strongly agree | 1 | 2 | 3 | 4 | 5 | strongly disagree |

If I begin to relapse, I will panic

| Strongly agree | 1 | 2 | 3 | 4 | 5 | strongly disagree |

If I begin to relapse, I will not make a fool of myself

| Strongly agree | 1 | 2 | 3 | 4 | 5 | strongly disagree |

If I begin to relapse, I will feel frightened that I will never be well again

| Strongly agree | 1 | 2 | 3 | 4 | 5 | strongly disagree |

If I begin to relapse, I will not lose my family and friends

| Strongly agree | 1 | 2 | 3 | 4 | 5 | strongly disagree |

If I begin to relapse, I will not lose control of myself

| Strongly agree | 1 | 2 | 3 | 4 | 5 | strongly disagree |

C. Control over relapse

No matter what I do, if I'm going to relapse, I will relapse

| Strongly agree | 1 | 2 | 3 | 4 | 5 | strongly disagree |

There are things I can do when I notice early signs to stop myself relapsing					
Strongly agree	1	2	3	4	5	strongly disagree

When I notice signs of relapsing, I ignore them					
Strongly agree	1	2	3	4	5	strongly disagree

I have learned to recognize my early signs of relapse (and know how to deal with them)					
Strongly agree	1	2	3	4	5	strongly disagree

I can't help panicking when I notice early signs of relapse					
Strongly agree	1	2	3	4	5	strongly disagree

When I begin to relapse, I enjoy the feelings too much to do anything about them					
Strongly agree	1	2	3	4	5	strongly disagree

Appendix 12: Relapse prevention plan

WHAT TO LOOK FOR	WHAT TO DO	
FIRST SIGNS	MYSELF	FAMILY/FRIENDS
MIDDLE SIGNS	MYSELF	FAMILY/FRIENDS
LATE SIGNS	MYSELF	FAMILY/FRIENDS

Appendix 13: Checklist of interventions completed

PHYSICAL ASSESSMENT AND PSYCHOSOCIAL FORMULATION

☐ Physical screening undertaken

☐ Diagrammatic CBT formulation completed   ☐ Young person given copy

☐ Formulation letter written collaboratively

PSYCHOEDUCATION

☐ Discussed explanatory model   ☐ Family

☐ Given verbal information   ☐ Family

☐ Given handouts   ☐ Family

☐ No medication option discussed   ☐ Family

INSIGHT/ADAPTATION

☐ Timeline

☐ Repertory grids

☐ Discussion around stigma

☐ First person accounts given

MEDICATION ADHERENCE

☐ Medication attitudes matrix

☐ Reasons assessed for potential non-adherence

☐ Reasons . . . .

☐ Involvement of significant others

☐ "Practical" solutions discussed (e.g. alarm or dosette box)

☐ "Psychological" solutions discussed (e.g. addressing stigma, psychoeducation, motivational interviewing)

☐ Health beliefs explored (attitudes and expectations)

CBT TECHNIQUES

☐ CBT format used (agenda, summary, homework, Socratic questioning)

☐ Reducing stimulation (mania/hypomania)/activity scheduling (depression)

☐ CBT rationale introduced

☐ Assessment of schemas

☐ Addressing unhelpful beliefs/schema work

☐ Behavioral experiments

SOCIAL RHYTHM

☐ Life events chart

☐ Assessment of daily routine

☐ Stress management work

☐ Encouragement of routine (sleep/exercise/diet)

FAMILY/RELATIONSHIPS

☐ Family debrief/support

☐ Confidentiality discussed

☐ Developmental/independence issues discussed

☐ Discussion of explanatory models

☐ Management of manic/depressed behavior

☐ Work to enhance communication

☐ Problem solving

COMORBIDITY

☐ Assessment of comorbidity

    ☐ Alcohol/drugs

    ☐ Anxiety/PTSD

    ☐ Abuse

    ☐ Other . . . .

☐ Anxiety management

☐ Motivational interviewing

RELAPSE PREVENTION

☐ Identification of early warning signs with copy for family/carers

☐ Identifying risk situations

☐ "Meaning" of relapse discussed

☐ Relapse plan (depression and mania)

☐ Letter to self

SOCIAL/OCCUPATIONAL FUNCTIONING

☐ Liaison with employment agency/employer/educational institution

☐ Support provided for return to work/study and/or maintenance of current work/study

☐ GOODBYE LETTER

ADDITIONAL INTERVENTIONS USED (list)

ADDITIONAL NOTES (e.g. why particular elements were not included)

References

Abou Jamra, R., Fuerst, R., Kaneva, R., et al. (2007). The First Genomewide Interaction and Locus-Heterogeneity Linkage Scan in Bipolar Affective Disorder: Strong Evidence of Epistatic Effects Between Loci on Chromosomes 2q and 6q. *American Journal of Human Genetics*, **81** (5), 974–86.

Ackerman, S. J., & Hilsenroth, M. J. (2003). A Review of Therapist Characteristics and Techniques Positively Impacting on the Therapeutic Alliance. *Clinical Psychology Review*, **23**, 1–33.

Agius, M., Oakham, H., Biocina, S. M., & Murphy, S. (2006). The Use of Card Sort Exercises in the Prevention of Relapse in Serious Mental Illness. *Psychiatria Danubina*, **18** (1–2), 61–73.

Allen, J. P., Litten, R. Z., Fertig, J. B., & Babor, T. (1997). A Review of Research on the Alcohol Use Disorders Identification Test (AUDIT). *Alcoholism: Clinical and Experimental Research*, **21** (4), 613–19.

Alloy, L. B., Abramson, L. Y., Urosevic, S., et al. (2005). The Psychosocial Context of Bipolar Disorder: Environmental, Cognitive and Developmental Risk Factors. *Clinical Psychology Review*, **25**, 1043–75.

Altman, S., Haeri S., Cohen L. J., et al. (2006). Predictors of Relapse in Bipolar Disorder: A Review. *Journal of Psychiatric Practice*, **12** (5), 269–82.

Amador, X. F., Flaum, M., Andreason, N., et al. (1994). Awareness of Illness in Schizophrenia and Schizoaffective and Mood Disorders. *Archives of General Psychiatry*, **51** (10), 826–36.

American Psychiatric Association (1994). *Diagnostic and Statistical Manual of Mental Disorders: Fourth Edition*. Washington, DC: American Psychiatric Association.

American Psychiatric Association (2000). *Diagnostic and Statistical Manual of Mental Disorders: Fourth Edition – Text Revision*. Washington, DC: American Psychiatric Association.

American Psychiatric Association (2002). *Practice Guidelines for the Treatment of Patients with Bipolar Disorder*. Arlington, VA: American Psychiatric Association.

Andrews, G., Creamer, M., Crino, R., et al. (2003). *The Treatment of Anxiety Disorders: Clinician Guides and Patient Treatment Manuals*. Cambridge: Cambridge University Press.

Angst, F., Stassen, H. H., Clayton, P. J., & Angst, J. (2002). Mortality of Patients with Mood Disorders: Follow Up over 34–38 Years. *Journal of Affective Disorders*, **68**, 167–81.

Angst, J. (2006). Do Many Patients with Depression Suffer from Bipolar Disorder? *Canadian Journal of Psychiatry*, **51** (1), 3–5.

Angst, J., & Marneros, A. (2001). Bipolarity from Ancient to Modern Times: Conception, Birth and Rebirth. *Journal of Affective Disorders*, **67**, 3–19.

Annis, H. M., Graham, J. M., & Davis, C. S. (1987). *Inventory of Drinking Situations (IDS-42)*. Toronto: Centre for Addiction and Mental Health.

Babiker, I. E. (1986). Non-Compliance in Schizophrenia. *Psychiatric Developments*, **4**, 329–37.

Babyak, M., Blumenthal, J. A., Herman, S., et al. (2000). Exercise Treatment for Major Depression: Maintenance of Therapeutic Benefit at 10 Months. *Psychosomatic Medicine*, **62** (5), 633–8.

Baldessarini, R. J., Tondo, L., & Hennen, J. (1999). Treatment Delays in Bipolar Disorders. *American Journal of Psychiatry*, **156** (5), 811–12.

Ball, J., Mitchell, P., Malhi, G., Skillecorn, A., & Smith, M. (2003). Schema-Focused Cognitive Therapy for Bipolar Disorder: Reducing Vulnerability to Relapse Through Attitudinal Change. *Australian and New Zealand Journal of Psychiatry*, **37**, 41–8.

Bateman, J. F., Agoston, T., Kovitz, B., & McCulloch, M. W. (1954). The Manic State as an Emergency Defense Reaction. *Journal of Nervous and Mental Diseases*, **119** (4), 349–57.

Bauer, M. S., & McBride, L. (2003). *Structured Group Psychotherapy for Bipolar Disorder: The Life Goals Program*, 2nd edn. New York: Springer Publishing Company.

Bauer, M., Unutzer, J., Pincus, H. A., & Lawson, W. B. (2002). Bipolar Disorder. *Mental Health Services Research*, **4** (4), 225–9.

Bebbington, P., Wilkins, S., Jones, P. B., et al. (1993). Life Events and Psychosis: Initial Results from the Camberwell Collaborative Psychosis Study. *British Journal of Psychiatry*, **162**, 72–9.

Beck, A. T. (1976). *Cognitive Therapy and the Emotional Disorders*. New York: Guilford Press.

Beck, A. T., Colis, M. J., Steer, R. A., Madrak, L., & Goldberg, J. F. (2006). Cognition Checklist for Mania-Revised. *Psychiatry Research*, **145** (2–3), 233–40.

Beck, A. T., Rush, A. J., Shaw, B. F., & Emery, G. (1979). *Cognitive Therapy of Depression*. New York: Guilford Press.

Begley, C. E., Annegers, J. F., Swann, A. C., et al. (2001). The Lifetime Cost of Bipolar Disorder in the U.S. *Pharmacoeconomics*, **19** (5 pt 1), 483–95.

Bennett, H. J. (2003). Humor in Medicine. *Southern Medical Journal*, **96** (12), 1257–61.

Bentall, R. (2003). *Madness Explained: Psychosis and Human Nature*. London: The Penguin Press.

Berk, M. (2007). Should we be Targeting Smoking as a Routine Intervention? *Acta Neuropsychiatrica*, **19** (2), 131–2.

Berk, M., Berk, L., & Castle, D. (2004). A Collaborative Approach to the Treatment Alliance in Bipolar Disorder. *Bipolar Disorders*, **6**, 504–18.

Berk, M., Dodd, S., Callaly, P., et al. (2007). History of Illness Prior to a Diagnosis of Bipolar Disorder or Schizoaffective Disorder. *Journal of Affective Disorders*, **103** (1–3), 181–6.

Berk, M., Dodd, S., Hallam, K., et al. (2008a). How Big a Shift in Diurnal Rhythms is Enough to be Clinically Relevant? A Naturalistic Study of Suicide and Daylight Saving. *Sleep and Biological Rhythms*, **6** (1), 22–5.

Berk, M., Ng, F., Wang, W. V., et al. (2008b). Going up in Smoke: Tobacco Smoking is Associated with Worse Treatment Outcomes in Mania. *Journal of Affective Disorders*, **110** (1–2), 126–34.

Berrettini, W. H. (2000). Susceptibility Loci for Bipolar Disorder: Overlap with Inherited Vulnerability to Schizophrenia. *Biological Psychiatry*, **47** (3), 245–51.

Berrettini, W. H., Ferraro, T. N., Goldin, L. R., et al. (1994). Chromosome 18 DNA Markers and Manic-Depressive Illness: Evidence for a Susceptibility Gene. *Proceedings of the National Academy of Sciences of the USA*, **91** (13), 5918–21.

Beynon, S., Soares-Weiser, K., Woolacott, N., Duffy, S., & Geddes, J. R. (2008). Psychosocial Interventions for the Prevention of Relapse in Bipolar Disorder: Systematic Review of Controlled Trials. *British Journal of Psychiatry*, **192**, 5–11.

Biederman, J., Birmaher, B., Carlson, G. A., et al. (2001). National Institute of Mental Health Research Roundtable on Prepubertal Bipolar Disorder. *Journal of the American Academy of Child and Adolescent Psychiatry*, **40** (8), 871–8.

Biederman, J., Faraone, S. V., Wozniak, J., (2005). Clinical Correlates of Bipolar Disorder in a Large, Referred Sample of Children and Adolescents. *Journal of Psychiatric Research*, **39**, 611–22.

Biukians, A., Miklowitz, D. J., & Kim, E. Y. (2007). Behavioral Activation, Inhibition and Mood Disorders in Early-Onset Bipolar Disorder. *Journal of Affective Disorders*, **97**, 71–6.

Blackburn, I. M., & Davidson, K. (1995). *Cognitive Therapy for Depression and Anxiety: A Practitioner's Guide*. Oxford: Blackwell Science.

Blairy, S., Linotte, S., Souery, D., et al. (2004). Social Adjustment and Self-Esteem of Bipolar Patients. *Journal of Affective Disorders*, **79**, 97–103.

Blatt, S. J., Sanislow, C. A., Zuroff, D. C., & Pilkonis, P. A. (1996). Characteristics of Effective Therapists: Further Analyses of Data From the National Institute of Mental Health Treatment of Depression Collaborative Research Program. *Journal of Consulting and Clinical Psychology*, **64** (6), 1276–84.

Boker, H., Hell, D., Budischewski, K., (2000). Personality and Object Relations in Patients with Affective Disorders: Idiographic Research by Means of the Repertory Grid Technique. *Journal of Affective Disorders*, **60**, 53–9.

Bowden, C. L. (2001). Strategies to Reduce Misdiagnosis of Bipolar Depression. *Psychiatric Services*, **52**(1), 51–55.

Brabban, A., & Turkington, D. (2002). The Search for Meaning: Detecting Congruence between Life Events, Underlying Schema and Psychotic Symptoms. In Morrison, A.P., ed., *A Casebook of Cognitive Therapy for Psychosis*, East Sussex: Brunner-Routledge, 59–75.

Brent, D. A., Kolko, D. J., Birmaher, B., et al. (1998). Predictors of Treatment Efficacy in a Clinical Trial of Three Psychosocial Treatments for Adolescent Depression. *Journal of the American Academy of Child and Adolescent Psychiatry*, **37** (9), 906–14.

British Psychological Society (2000). *Recent Advances in Understanding Mental Illness and Psychotic Experience*. Leicester: British Psychological Society.

Brown, G. K., Beck, A. T., Steer, R. A., & Grisham, J. R. (2000). Risk Factors for Suicide in Psychiatric Outpatients: A 20-Year Prospective Study. *Journal of Consulting and Clinical Psychology*, **68** (3), 371–7.

Burke, K. C., Burke, J. D., Regier, D. A., & Rae, D. S. (1990). Age at Onset of Selected Mental Disorders in Five Community Populations. *Archives of General Psychiatry*, **47**, 511–18.

Cade, J. F. J. (1949). Lithium Salts in the Treatment of Manic Excitement. *The Medical Journal of Australia*, **36**, 349–52.

Calhoun, L. G., & Tedeschi, R. G. (1999). *Facilitating Posttraumatic Growth: A Clinician's Guide*. London: Erlbaum.

Carlson, G. A. (1985). Bipolar Disorder in Adolescence. *Psychiatric Annals*, **15** (6), 379–86.

Carlson, G. A., Bromet, E. J., & Sievers, S. (2000). Phenomenology and Outcome of Subjects with Early and Adult Onset Psychotic Mania. *American Journal of Psychiatry*, **157** (2), 213–19.

Cassidy, F., McEvoy, J. P., Yang, Y. K., & Wilson, W. H. (2001). Insight is Greater in Mixed than in Pure Manic Episodes of Bipolar I Disorder. *Journal of Nervous and Mental Disease*, **189** (6), 398–9.

Castonguay, L. G., Goldfried, M. R., Wiser, S., Raue, P. J., & Hayes, A. M. (1996). Predicting the Effect of Cognitive Therapy for Depression: A Study of Unique and Common Factors. *Journal of Consulting and Clinical Psychology*, **64** (3), 497–504.

Chadwick, P., Birchwood, M., & Trower, P. (1996). *Cognitive Therapy for Delusions, Voices and Paranoia*. West Sussex: John Wiley & Sons, Ltd.

Chen, Y. W., & Dilsaver, S. C. (1996). Lifetime Rates of Suicide Attempts among Subjects with Bipolar and Unipolar Disorders Relative to Subjects with Other Axis I Disorders. *Biological Psychiatry*, **39** (10), 896–9.

Cochran, S. D. (1984). Preventing Medical Noncompliance in the Outpatient Treatment of Bipolar Affective Disorders. *Journal of Consulting and Clinical Psychology*, **52**, 873–8.

Coletti, D. J., Leigh, E., Gallelli, K. A., & Kafantaris, V. (2005). Patterns of Adherence to Treatment in Adolescents with Bipolar Disorder. *Journal of Child and Adolescent Psychopharmacology*, **15**, 913–17.

Colom, F. (2006). *Psychoeducation Manual for Bipolar Disorder*. Cambridge: Cambridge University Press.

Colom, F. (2008). Long-Term Follow Up of Psychotherapies in Bipolar Disorder. *Bipolar Disorders*, **10** (Suppl. 1), 20.

Colom, F., Vieta, E., Martinez-Aran, A., et al. (2003). A Randomized Trial on the Efficacy of Group Psychoeducation in the Prophylaxis of Recurrences in Bipolar Patients whose Disease is in Remission. *Archives of General Psychiatry*, **60** (4), 402–7.

Colom, F., Vieta, E., Tacchi, M. J., Sanchez-Moreno, J., & Scott, J. (2005). Identifying and Improving Non-Adherence in Bipolar Disorders. *Bipolar Disorders*, **7** (Suppl. 5), 24–31.

Colombo, C., Benedetti, F., Barbini, B., Campori, E., & Smeraldi, E. (1999). Rate of Switch from Depression into Mania after Therapeutic Sleep Deprivation in Bipolar Depression. *Psychiatry Research*, **86**, 267–70.

Conus, P., Cotton, S., Abdel-Baki, A., et al. (2006). Symptomatic and Functional Outcome 12 Months after a First Episode of Psychotic Mania: Barriers to Recovery in a Catchment Area Sample. *Bipolar Disorders*, **8** (3), 221–31.

Conus, P., Cotton, S., Graf-Schimmelmann, B., McGorry, P. D., & Lambert, M. (2007). The First-Episode Psychosis Outcome Study: Premorbid and Baseline Characteristics of an Epidemiological Cohort of 661 First-Episode Psychosis Patients. *Early Intervention in Psychiatry*, **1**, 191–200.

Conus, P., & McGorry, P. D. (2002). First Episode Mania: A Neglected Priority for Early Intervention. *Australian and New Zealand Journal of Psychiatry*, **36**, 158–72.

Corsano, P., Majorano, M., & Champretavy, L. (2006). Psychological Well-Being in Adolescence: The Contribution of Interpersonal Relationships and Experience of Being Alone. *Adolescence*, **41** (162), 341–53.

Coryell, W., Endicott, J., Andreason, N., & Keller, M. (1985). Bipolar I, Bipolar II and Non-Bipolar Major Depression among Relatives of Affectively Ill Probands. *American Journal of Psychiatry*, **142**, 817–21.

Coryell, W., Scheftner, W., Keller, M., et al. (1993). The Enduring Psychosocial Consequences of Mania and Depression. *American Journal of Psychiatry*, **150** (5), 720–7.

Coryell, W., Solomon, D., Leon, A. C., et al. (1998). Lithium Discontinuation and Subsequent Effectiveness. *American Journal of Psychiatry*, **155** (7), 895–8.

Cramer, J. A., & Rosenheck, R. (1998). Compliance with Medication Regimens for Mental and Physical Disorders. *Psychiatric Services*, **49** (2), 196–201.

Crits-Cristoph, P., Baranackie, K., Kurcias, J. S., et al. (1991). Meta-Analysis of Therapist Effects in Psychotherapy Outcome Studies. *Psychotherapy Research*, **1**, 81–91.

Cummings, C., Gordon, J., & Marlatt, G. (1980). Relapse: Prevention and Prediction. In Miller, W., ed., *The Addictive Behaviours: Treatment of Alcoholism, Drug Abuse, Smoking and Obesity*. Oxford: Pergamon Press.

Curry, J. F. (2001). Specific Psychotherapies for Childhood and Adolescent Depression. *Biological Psychiatry*, **49**, 1091–100.

Danielson, C. K., Feeny, N. C., Findling, R. L., & Youngstrom, E. A. (2004). Psychosocial Treatment of Bipolar Disorders in Adolescents: A Proposed Cognitive-Behavioral Intervention. *Cognitive and Behavioral Practice*, **11**, 283–97.

Davidson, K. (2000). *Cognitive Therapy for Personality Disorders*. London: Arnold.

Davidson, K., & Scott, J. (2008). Therapist Competency in Psychotherapy. *Psychiatric Bulletin*, in press.

Davies, E. The Attitude to Relapse Scale. Unpublished doctoral dissertation, The University of Birmingham.

Dell'Osso, L., Pini, S., Mastrocinque, C., et al. (2002). Insight into Illness in Patients with Mania, Mixed Mania, Bipolar Depression and Major Depression with Psychotic Features. *Bipolar Disorders*, **4** (5), 315–22.

Diamond, D., & Doane, J. A. (1994). Disturbed Attachment and Negative Affect Style: An Intergenerational Spiral. *British Journal of Psychiatry*, **164**, 770–81.

Dooley, L. (1921). A Psychoanalytic Study of Manic Depressive Psychosis. *Psychoanalytic Review*, **8**, 38–72.

Drotar, D., Greenley, R. N., Demeter, C. A., et al. (2007). Adherence to Pharmacological Treatment for Juvenile Bipolar Disorder. *Journal of the American Academy of Child and Adolescent Psychiatry*, **46** (7), 831–9.

Dumont, M., & Provost, M. A. (1999). Resilience in Adolescents: Protective Role of Social Support, Coping Strategies, Self-Esteem, and Social Activities on Experience of Stress and Depression. *Journal of Youth and Adolescence*, **28** (3), 343–63.

Dunkley, J. E., Bates, G., Foulds, M., & Fitzgerald, P. (2007). Understanding Adaptation to First-Episode Psychosis: The Relevance of Trauma and Posttraumatic Growth. *The Australasian Journal of Disaster and Trauma Studies*, **1**, 1–17.

Egeland, J. A., Hostetter, A. M., Pauls, D. L., & Sussex, J. N. (2000). Prodromal Symptoms Before Onset of Manic-Depressive Disorder Suggested by First Hospital Admission Histories. *Journal of the American Academy of Child and Adolescent Psychiatry*, **39** (10), 1245–52.

Eich, E., Macauley, D., & Ryan, L. (1994). Mood Dependent Memory for Events in the Personal Past. *Journal of Experimental Psychology*, **123**, 201–15.

Eisenthal, S., Emery, R., Lazare, A., & Udin, H. (1979). Adherence and the Negotiated Approach to Patienthood. *Archives of General Psychiatry*, **36**, 393–8.

Elgie, R., & Morselli, P. L. (2007). Social Functioning in Bipolar Patients: The Perception and Perspective of Patients, Relatives and Advocacy Organizations – a Review. *Bipolar Disorders*, **9**, 144–57.

Ellicott, A., Hammen, C., Gitlin, M., Brown G., & Jamison, K. (1990). Life Events and the Course of Bipolar Disorder. *American Journal of Psychiatry*, **147**, 1194–8.

Ellis, N., Crone, D., Davey, R., & Grogan, S. (2007). Exercise Interventions as an Adjunct Therapy for Psychosis: A Critical Review. *British Journal of Clinical Psychology*, **46** (1), 95–111.

Erickson, M. H., & Rossi, E. L. (1979). *Experiencing Hypnosis: Therapeutic Approaches to Altered States*. New York: Irvington.

Ernst, C. L., & Goldberg, J. F. (2004). Clinical Features Related to Age at Onset in Bipolar Disorder. *Journal of Affective Disorders*, **82**, 21–7.

Evans, J., Heron, J., Lewis, G., Araya, R., & Wolke, D. (2005). Negative Self-Schemas and the Onset of Depression in Women: Longitudinal Study. *British Journal of Psychiatry*, **186**, 302–7.

Evans, K., McGrath, J., & Milns, R. (2003). Searching for Schizophrenia in Ancient Greek and Roman Literature: A Systematic Review. *Acta Psychiatrica Scandinavica*, **107**, 323–30.

Feeny, N. C., Danielson, C. K., Schwartz, L., Youngstrom, E. A., & Findling, R. L. (2006). Cognitive-Behavioral Therapy for Bipolar Disorders in Adolescents: A Pilot Study. *Bipolar Disorders*, **8**, 508–15.

Fennell, M. (1989). Depression. In Hawton, K., Salkovskis, P. M., Kirk, J., & Clark, D. M., eds., *Cognitive Behavioural Therapy for Psychiatric Problems: A Practical Guide*. Oxford: Oxford University Press.

Festinger, L. (1957). *A Theory of Cognitive Dissonance*. Palo Alto, California: Stanford University Press.

Fox, S., Rainie, L., Horrigan, J., et al. (2000). *The Online Healthcare Revolution: How the Web Helps Americans Take Better Care of Themselves*. Washington, DC: Pew Internet & American Life Project.

Francis-Raniere, E. L., Alloy, L. B., & Abramson, L. Y. (2006). Depressive Personality Styles and Bipolar Spectrum Disorders: Prospective Tests of the Event Congruency Hypothesis. *Bipolar Disorders*, **8**, 382–99.

Frank, A. F., & Gunderson, J. G. (1990). The Role of the Therapeutic Alliance in the Treatment of Schizophrenia. *Archives of General Psychiatry*, **47**, 228–36.

Frank, E. (2007). *Treating Bipolar Disorder: A Clinician's Guide to Interpersonal and Social Rhythm Therapy*. New York: Guilford Press.

Frank, E., Kupfer, D. J., Thase, M. E., et al. (2005). Two-Year Outcomes for Interpersonal and Social Rhythm Therapy for Individuals with Bipolar I Disorder. *Archives of General Psychiatry*, **62**, 996–1004.

Frank, E., Schwarz, H. A., & Kupfer, D. J. (2000). Interpersonal and Social Rhythm Therapy: Managing the Chaos of Bipolar Disorder. *Biological Psychiatry*, **48**, 593–604.

Freud, S. (1921). Group Psychotherapy and the Analysis of the Ego. In Strachey, J., ed., *The Complete Psychological Works of Sigmund Freud* (Vol. 18). London: Hogarth Press, 132–3.

Frey, B. N., Andreazza, A. C., Nery, F. G., et al. (2007). The Role of Hippocampus in the Pathophysiology of Bipolar Disorder. *Behavioural Pharmacology*, **18** (5–6), 419–30.

Garland, A., & Scott, J. (2002). Using Homework in Therapy for Depression. *Journal of Clinical Psychology*, **58**, 489–98.

Gaston, L. (1991). Reliability and Criterion-Related Validity of the California Psychotherapy Alliance Scales – Patient Version. *Psychological Assessment*, **3**, 68–74.

Gelenberg, A. J., Kane, J. N., Keller, M. B., et al. (1989). Comparison of Standard and Low Serum Levels of Lithium for Maintenance Treatment of Bipolar Disorders. *New England Journal of Medicine*, **321**, 1489–93.

Geller, B., Craney, J. L., Bolhofner, K., et al. (2002). Two-Year Prospective Follow-Up of Children with a Prepubertal and Early Adolescent Bipolar Disorder Phenotype. *American Journal of Psychiatry*, **159**, 927–33.

Ghaemi, S. N., Boiman, E. E., & Goodwin, F. K. (2000a). Diagnosing Bipolar Disorder and the Effect of Antidepressants: Naturalistic Study. *Journal of Clinical Psychiatry*, **61**, 804–8.

Ghaemi, S. N., Boiman, E. E., & Goodwin, F. K. (2000b). Insight and Outcome in Bipolar, Unipolar, and Anxiety Disorders. *Comprehensive Psychiatry*, **41** (3), 167–71.

Ghaemi, S. N., Ko, J. Y., & Goodwin, F. K. (2002). Cade's Disease and Beyond: Misdiagnosis, Antidepressant Use and a Proposed Definition for Bipolar Spectrum Disorder. *Canadian Journal of Psychiatry*, **47**, 125–34.

Gilbert, P. (2000). *Overcoming Depression: A Self Help Guide Using Cognitive Behavioural Techniques*. London: Constable & Robinson Ltd.

Ginsberg, G. L. (1979). Psychoanalytic Aspects of Mania. In Shopsin, B., ed., *Manic Illness*. New York: Raven Press.

Gitlin, M. J., Swendson, J., Heller, T. L., & Hammen C. (1995). Relapse and Impairment in Bipolar Disorder. *American Journal of Psychiatry*, **152**, 1635–49.

Glaser, N., Kazantzis, N., Deane, F. P., & Oades, L. G. (2000). Critical Issues in Using Homework Assignments within Cognitive-Behavioral Therapy for Schizophrenia. *Journal of Rational-Emotive and Cognitive-Behavior Therapy*, **18** (4), 247–61.

Goldberg, J. F., Wenze, S. J., Welker, T. M., Steer, R. A., & Beck, A. T. (2005). Content-Specificity of Dysfunctional Cognitions for Patients with Bipolar Mania versus Unipolar Depression: A Preliminary Study. *Bipolar Disorders*, **7**, 49–56.

Goldstein, T. R., Miklowitz, D. J., & Richards, J. A. (2002). Expressed Emotion Attitudes and Individual Psychopathology Among the Relatives of Bipolar Patients. *Family Process*, **41** (4), 645–57.

Golombek, H., Marton, P., Stein, B. A., & Korenblum, M. (1989). Adolescent Personality Development: Three Phases, Three Courses and Varying Turmoil. Findings from the Toronto Adolescent Longitudinal Study. *Canadian Journal of Psychiatry*, **34**, 500–4.

Gonzalez-Pinto, A., Gonzalez, C., Enjuto, S., et al. (2004). Psychoeducation and Cognitive-Behavioral Therapy in Bipolar Disorder: An Update. *Acta Psychiatrica Scandinavica*, **109**, 83–90.

Goodwin, F., & Jamison, K. (1990). *Manic Depressive Illness*. Oxford: Oxford University Press.

Goodwin, F., & Jamison, K. (2007). *Manic Depressive Illness: Bipolar Disorders and Recurrent Depression*, 2nd edn. Oxford: Oxford University Press.

Gordon, J., & Grant, G., eds. (1997). *How We Feel: An Insight into the Emotional World of Teenagers*. London: Jessica Kingsley Publishers.

Graf-Schimmelmann, B., Conus, P., Schacht, M., McGorry, P., & Lambert, M. (2006). Predictors of Service Disengagement in First Admitted Adolescents with Psychosis. *Journal of the American Academy of Child and Adolescent Psychiatry*, **45** (8), 990–9.

Granek-Catarivas, M., Goldstein-Ferber, S., Azuri, Y., & Kahan, E. (2006). Use of Humour in Primary Care: Different Perceptions Among Patients and Physicians. *Postgraduate Medical Journal*, **81**, 126–30.

Greenhouse, W. J., Meyer, B., & Johnson, S. L. (2000). Coping and Medication Adherence in Bipolar Disorder. *Journal of Affective Disorders*, **59**, 237–41.

Gumley, A., Karantzias, A., Power, K., et al. (2006). Early Intervention for Relapse in Schizophrenia: Impact of Cognitive Behavioural Therapy on Negative Beliefs about Psychosis and Self-Esteem. *British Journal of Clinical Psychology*, **45** (2), 247–60.

Gumley, A., & Schwannauer, M. (2006). *Staying Well After Psychosis: A Cognitive Interpersonal Approach to Recovery and Relapse Prevention*. West Sussex: John Wiley & Sons, Ltd.

Gumley, A., White, C. A., & Power, K. (1999). An Interacting Cognitive Subsystems Model of Relapse and the Course of Psychosis. *Clinical Psychology and Psychotherapy*, **6** (4), 261–78.

Guscott, R., & Taylor, L. (1994). Lithium Prophylaxis in Recurrent Affective Illness. Efficacy, Effectiveness and Efficiency. *British Journal of Psychiatry*, **164** (6), 741–6.

Haidt, J. (2006). *The Happiness Hypothesis*. London: Arrow Books.

Hamilton, T. K., & Schweitzer, R. D. (2000). The Cost of Being Perfect: Perfectionism and Suicide Ideation in University Students. *Australian and New Zealand Journal of Psychiatry*, **34**, 829–35.

Hammen, C., & Gitlin, M. (1997). Stress Reactivity in Bipolar Patients and its Relation to Prior History of Disorder. *American Journal of Psychiatry*, **154**, 856–7.

Harvey, A. (2000). Sleep Hygiene and Sleep-Onset Insomnia. *The Journal of Nervous and Mental Disease*, **188** (1), 53–5.

Hasty, M. K., Macneil, C. A., Kader, L. F., et al. (2006). *The Developmental Considerations for Psychological Treatment of First Episode Bipolar Disorder*. 5th International Conference on Early Psychosis, Birmingham, England.

Haynes, R. B. (1976). A Critical Review of the "Determinants" of Patient Compliance with Therapeutic Regimens. In Sackett, D. L., & Haynes, R. B., eds., *Compliance with Therapeutic Regimens*. Baltimore: Johns Hopkins University Press.

Hayward, P., Wong, G., Bright, J. A., & Lam, D. (2002). Stigma and Self Esteem in Manic Depression: An Exploratory Study. *Journal of Affective Disorders*, **69**, 61–7.

Healy, D., & Williams, J. (1989). Moods, Misattributions and Mania. *Psychiatric Developments*, **1**, 49–70.

Heider, D., Bernert, S., Matschinger, H., et al. (2007). Parental Bonding and Suicidality in Adulthood. *Australian and New Zealand Journal of Psychiatry*, **41**, 66–73.

Heider, D., Matschinger, H., Bernert, S., Alonso, J., & Angermeyer, M. C. (2006). Relationship Between Parental Bonding and Mood Disorder in Six European Countries. *Psychiatry Research*, **143** (1), 89–98.

Henry, L., Edwards, J., Jackson, H., Hulbert, C., & McGorry, P. (2002). *Cognitively Oriented Psychotherapy for First-Episode Psychosis (COPE): A Practitioner's Manual*. Victoria, Australia: EPPIC.

Hill, J. (1983). Early Adolescence: A Research Agenda. *Journal of Early Adolescence*, **3**, 1–21.

Hilty, D. M., Brady, K. T., & Hales, R. E. (1999). A Review of Bipolar Disorder Among Adults. *Psychiatric Services*, **50** (2), 201–13.

Hinton, M., Elkins, K., Edwards, J., & Donovan, K. (2002). *Cannabis and Psychosis: An Early Psychosis Treatment Manual*. Melbourne, Victoria: Government of Victoria, Department of Human Services.

Hirschfeld, R. M., Lewis, L., & Vornik, L. A. (2003). Perceptions and Impact of Bipolar Disorder: How Far Have we Really Come? Results of the National Depressive and Manic Depressive Association 2000 Survey of Individuals with Bipolar Disorder. *Journal of Clinical Psychiatry*, **64**, 161–74.

Hlastala, S., & Frank, E. (2006). Adapting Interpersonal and Social Rhythm Therapy to the Developmental Needs of Adolescents with Bipolar Disorder. *Development and Psychopathology*, **18**, 1267–88.

Hlastala, S., Frank, E., Kowalski, J., et al. (2000). Stressful Life Events, Bipolar Disorder and the "Kindling Model." *Journal of Abnormal Psychology*, **109**, 777–86.

Homer (2007). *The Odyssey*. Raleigh, North Carolina: Hayes Barton Press, Vitalsource Technologies.

Horvath, A. O., & Greenberg, L. S. (1989). Development and Validation of the Working Alliance Inventory. *Journal of Counseling Psychology*, **36** (2), 223–33.

Huxley, N. A., Parikh, S. V., & Baldessarini, R. J. (2000). Effectiveness of Psychosocial Treatments in Bipolar Disorder: State of the Evidence. *Harvard Review of Psychiatry*, **8** (3), 126–40.

Hyman, S. E. (1999). Introduction to the Complex Genetics of Mental Disorders. *Biological Psychiatry*, **45** (5), 518–21.

Jackson, A., Cavanagh, J., & Scott, J. (2003). A Systematic Review of Manic and Depressive Prodromes. *Journal of Affective Disorders*, **74**, 209–17.

Jackson, H. J., Edwards, J., Hulbert, C., & McGorry, P. D. (1999). Recovery from Psychosis: Psychological Interventions. In McGorry, P. D., & Jackson, H. J., eds., *The Recognition and Management of Early Psychosis: A Preventive Approach*. Cambridge: Cambridge University Press.

James A., Soler A., & Weatherall, R. (2005). Cognitive Behavioural Therapy for Anxiety Disorders in Children and Adolescents. *Cochrane Database of Systematic Reviews*, (4), CD004690.

Jamison, K. R. (1995). *An Unquiet Mind: A Memoir of Moods and Madness*. Oxford: Picador.

Jamison, K. R. (2003). Foreword. In Power, M., ed., *A Handbook of Science and Practice: Mood Disorders*. West Sussex: John Wiley & Sons, Ltd.

Jamison, K. R., & Akiskal, H. S. (1983). Medication Compliance in Patients with Bipolar Disorder. *Psychiatric Clinics of North America*, **6** (1), 175–92.

Joffe, R. T., MacQueen, G. M., Marriott, M., & Young, L. T. (2004). A Prospective, Longitudinal Study of Percentage of Time Spent Ill in Patients with Bipolar I or Bipolar II Disorders. *Bipolar Disorders*, **6**, 62–6.

Johnson, R. C. (1996). The Wonder-Rabbi of Kuzmir as a Behaviour Therapist. *Behavioural and Cognitive Psychotherapy*, 24, 367–70.

Johnson, R., & McFarland, B. (1996). Lithium Use and Discontinuation in a Health Maintenance Organization. *American Journal of Psychiatry*, 153, 993–1000.

Johnson, S. L. (2005). Mania and Dysregulation in Goal Pursuit: A Review. *Clinical Psychology Review*, 25, 241–62.

Johnson, S. L., & Leahy, R. L. (2004). *Psychological Treatment of Bipolar Disorder*. New York: Guilford Press.

Johnson, S. L., Sandrow, D., Meyer, B., et al. (2000). Increases in Manic Symptoms after Life Events Involving Goal Attainment. *Journal of Abnormal Psychology*, 4, 721–7.

Jones, L., Scott, J., Haque, S., et al. (2005b). Cognitive Style in Bipolar Disorder. *British Journal of Psychiatry*, 187, 431–7.

Jones, S. (2004). Psychotherapy of Bipolar Disorder: A Review. *Journal of Affective Disorders*, 80, 101–14.

Jones, S., Hayward, P., & Lam, D. (2002). *Coping with Bipolar Disorder: A Guide to Living with Manic Depression*. Oxford: Oneworld Publications.

Jones, S. H., Sellwood, W., & McGovern, J. (2005a). Psychological Therapies for Bipolar Disorder: The Role of Model-Driven Approaches to Therapy Integration. *Bipolar Disorders*, 7, 22–32.

Jones, S. H., & Tarrier, N. (2005). New Developments in Bipolar Disorder (Editorial). *Clinical Psychology Review*, 25, 1003–7.

Joseph, S., & Linley, P. A. (2004). Growth Following Adversity: Theoretical Perspectives and Implications for Clinical Practice. *Clinical Psychology Review*, 26, 1041–53.

Judd, L. L., Akiskal, H. S., Schettler, P. J., et al. (2002). The Long Term Natural History of the Weekly Symptomatic Status of Bipolar I Disorder. *Archives of General Psychiatry*, 59 (6), 530–7.

Kahn, D. (1990). The Psychotherapy of Mania. *Psychiatric Clinics of North America*, 13 (2), 229–40.

Kato, T. (2007). Molecular Genetics of Bipolar Disorder and Depression. *Psychiatry and Clinical Neurosciences*, 61, 3–19.

Kazantzis, N., Deane, F. P., & Ronan, K. R. (2000). Homework Assignments in Cognitive and Behavioral Therapy: A Meta-Analysis. *Clinical Psychology: Science and Practice*, 7 (2), 189–202.

Keck, P. E., McElroy, S. L., Strakowski, S. M., et al. (1998). 12-Month Outcome of Patients with Bipolar Disorder Following Hospitalization for a Manic or Mixed Episode. *American Journal of Psychiatry*, 155 (5), 646–52.

Keijsers, G. P. J., Schaap, C. P. D. R., & Hoogduin, C. A. L. (2000). The Impact of Interpersonal Patient and Therapist Behavior on Outcome in Cognitive Behavior Therapy. *Behavior Modification*, 24 (2), 264–97.

Keller, M. B., Lavori, P. W., Coryell, W., Endicott, J., & Mueller, T. I. (1993). Bipolar I: A Five-Year Prospective Follow-Up. *Journal of Nervous and Mental Disease*, 181 (4), 238–45.

Kelly, G. (1955). *The Psychology of Personal Constructs*. New York: Norton.

Kennedy, S., Thompson, R., Stancer, H. C., Roy, A., & Persad, E. (1983). Life Events Precipitating Mania. *British Journal of Psychiatry*, 142, 398–403.

Kernis, M. H., Cornell, D. P., Sun, C. R., Berry, A., & Harlow, T. (1993). There's More to Self-Esteem Than Whether it is High or Low: The Importance of Stability of Self-Esteem. *Journal of Personality and Social Psychology*, 61, 80–4.

Kessing, L. V. (1998). Recurrence in Affective Disorder: II. Effect of Age and Gender. *British Journal of Psychiatry*, 172, 29–34.

Kessing, L. V., Agerbo, E., & Mortensen, P. B. (2004). Major Life Events and Other Risk Factors for First Admission with Mania. *Bipolar Disorders*, 6, 122–9.

Kessler, R. C., McGonagle, K. A., Zhao, S., et al. (1994). Lifetime and 12 Month Prevalence of DSM IIIR Psychiatric Disorder in the United States. *Archives of General Psychiatry*, 51, 8–19.

Kestenbaum, C. J. (1982). Children and Adolescents at Risk for Manic-Depressive Illness: Introduction and Overview. *Adolescent Psychiatry*, 10, 245–55.

Klein, H. S. (1974). Transference and Defence in Manic States. *International Journal of Psycho-Analysis*, 55, 261–8.

Klerman, G. L., Olfson, M., Leon, A., & Weissman, M. M. (1992). Measuring the Need for Mental Health Care. *Health Affairs*, 11, 23–33.

Kohn, R., Saxena, S., Levav, I., & Saraceno, B. (2004). The Treatment Gap in Mental Health Care. *Bulletin of the World Health Organization*, 82 (11), 858–66.

Kottler, J. A. (2003). *On Being a Therapist*, 3rd edn. San Francisco: Jossey-Bass Publishers.

Kramer, S. A. (1990). *Positive Endings in Psychotherapy: Bringing Meaningful Closure to Therapeutic Relationships*. San Francisco: Jossey-Bass Publishers.

Kubler-Ross, E. (1970). *On Death and Dying*. New York: Collier Books/Macmillan Publishing Co.

Lally, S. J. (1989). Does Being in Here Mean There is Something Wrong with Me? *Schizophrenia Bulletin*, 15, 253–65.

Lam, D. (2006). What Can We Conclude from Studies on Psychotherapy in Bipolar Disorder? *British Journal of Psychiatry*, 188, 321–2.

Lam, D., Hayward, P., Watkins, E. R., Wright, K., & Sham, P. (2005). Relapse Prevention in Patients with Bipolar Disorders: Cognitive Therapy Outcome after 2 Years. *American Journal of Psychiatry*, 162 (2), 324–9.

Lam, D. H., Jones, S. H., Hayward, P., & Bright, J. A. (1999). *Cognitive Therapy for Bipolar Disorder: A Therapist's Guide to Concepts, Methods and Practice*. West Sussex: John Wiley & Sons, Ltd.

Lam D., & Wong, G. (2005). Prodromes, Coping Strategies and Psychological Interventions in Bipolar Disorders. *Clinical Psychology Review*, 25 (8), 1028–42.

Lam, D., Wright, K., & Smith, N. (2004). Dysfunctional Assumptions in Bipolar Disorder. *Journal of Affective Disorders*, 79, 193–9.

Lawlor, D. A., & Hopker, S. W. (2001). The Effect of Exercise as an Intervention in the Management of Depression: Systematic Review and Meta-Regression Analysis of Randomised Controlled Trials. *British Medical Journal*, 322, 763–7.

Leahy, R. L. (2001). *Overcoming Resistance in Cognitive Therapy*. New York: Guilford Press.

Leboyer, M., Henry, C., Paillere-Martinot, M. L., & Bellivier, F. (2005). Age at Onset in Bipolar Affective Disorders: A Review. *Bipolar Disorders*, 7, 111–18.

LeDoux, J. E. (1996). *The Emotional Brain: The Mysterious Underpinnings of Emotional Life*. New York: Simon & Schuster.

Leverich, G. S., & Post, R. M. (2006). Course of Bipolar Illness After History of Childhood Trauma. *Lancet*, 367, 1040–2.

Levinson, W., Roter, D. L., Mullooly, J. P., Dull, V. T., & Frankel, R. M. (1997). Physician-Patient Communication: The Relationship With Malpractice Claims among Primary Care Physicians and Surgeons. *Journal of the American Medical Association*, 277 (7), 553–9.

Lewinsohn, P. M., Seeley, J. R., & Klein, D. N. (2003). Bipolar Disorders During Adolescence. *Acta Psychiatrica Scandinavica*, 108 (Suppl. 418), 47–50.

Lewis, L. (2005). Patient Perspectives on the Diagnosis, Treatment and Management of Bipolar Disorder. *Bipolar Disorders*, 7 (Suppl. 1), 33–7.

Lingam, R., & Scott, J. (2002). Treatment Non-Adherence in Affective Disorders. *Acta Psychiatrica Scandinavica*, 105, 164–72.

Lingjaerde, O., Ahlfors, U., Bech, P., Dencker, S., & Elgen, K. (1987). The UKU Side Effect Rating Scale. *Acta Psychiatrica Scandinavica*, 76 (Suppl. 334), 1–100.

Lipkovich, I., Citrome, L., Perlis, R., et al. (2006). Early Predictors of Substantial Weight Gain in Bipolar Patients Treated with Olanzapine. *Journal of Clinical Psychopharmacology*, 26 (3), 316–20.

Lish, J. D., Dime-Meehan, S., Whybrow, P. C., Price, R. A., & Hirschfeld, R. M. (1994). The National Depressive and Manic Depressive Association (NMDA) Survey of Bipolar Members. *Journal of Affective Disorders*, 31, 281–94.

Lyon, H. M., Startup, M., & Bentall, R. P. (1999). Social Cognition and the Manic Defence: Attributions, Selective Attention, and Self-Schema in Bipolar Affective Disorder. *Journal of Abnormal Psychology*, **108** (2), 273–82.

Malhi, G. S., Lagopolous, J., Sachdev, P., et al. (2004). Cognitive Generation of Affect in Hypomania: An fMRI Study. *Bipolar Disorders*, **6**, 271–85.

Malkoff-Schwartz, S., Frank, E., Anderson, B., et al. (1998). Stressful Life Events and Social Rhythm Disruption in the Onset of Manic and Depressive Bipolar Episodes. *Archives of General Psychiatry*, **55**, 702–7.

Mansell, W., Colom, F., & Scott, J. (2005). The Nature and Treatment of Depression in Bipolar Disorder: A Review and Implications for Future Psychological Investigation. *Clinical Psychology Review*, **25** (8), 1076–100.

Mansell, W., & Lam, D. (2004). A Preliminary Study on Autobiographical Memory in Remitted Bipolar and Unipolar Depression and the Role of Imagery in the Specificity of Memory. *Memory*, **12** (4), 437–46.

Mansell, W., & Lam, D. (2006). "I Won't Do What You Tell Me!": Elevated Mood and the Assessment of Advice-Taking in Euthymic Bipolar I Disorder. *Behaviour Research and Therapy*, **44**, 1787–801.

Marneros, A., & Goodwin, F. K., eds. (2005). *Bipolar Disorders: Mixed States, Rapid Cycling and Atypical Forms*. Cambridge: Cambridge University Press.

Martinez-Aran, A., Vieta, E., Torrent, C., et al. (2007). Functional Outcome in Bipolar Disorders: The Role of Clinical and Cognitive Factors. *Bipolar Disorders*, **9**, 103–13.

Maslow, A. H. (1943). A Theory of Human Motivation. *Psychological Review*, **50** (4), 370–96.

Mason, O., Platts, H., & Tyson, M. (2005). Early Maladaptive Schemas and Adult Attachment in a UK Clinical Population. *Psychology and Psychotherapy*, **78**, 549–64.

May, R. (2004). Making Sense of Psychotic Experience and Working Towards Recovery. In Gleeson, J. F. M., & McGorry, P. D., eds., *Psychological Interventions in Early Psychosis: A Treatment Manual*. West Sussex: John Wiley & Sons, Ltd.

McElroy, S. L., Strakowski S. M., West S. A., Keck, P. E. Jr., & McConville, B. J. (1997). Phenomenology of Adolescent and Adult Mania in Hospitalized Patients with Bipolar Disorder. *American Journal of Psychiatry*, **154**, 44–9.

McEvoy, J. P., Apperson, L. J., Applebaum, P. S., et al. (1989). Insight in Schizophrenia: Its Relationship to Acute Psychopathology. *Journal of Nervous and Mental Disease*, **177**, 43–7.

McGlashan, T. H., & Carpenter, W. T. (1976). Post Psychotic Depression in Schizophrenia. *Archives of General Psychiatry*, **33**, 231–9.

McGlashan, T. H., Heinssen, R. K., & Fenton, W. S. (1990). Psychosocial Treatment of Negative Symptoms in Schizophrenia. In Andreasen, N. C., ed., *Modern Problems in Pharmacopsychiatry. Vol 24 Schizophrenia: Positive and Negative Symptoms and Syndromes*. Basel: Karger, 175–200.

McGoldrick, M., Gerson, R., & Petry, S. (2008). *Genograms: Assessment and Intervention*, 3rd edn. New York: Norton.

McGorry, P. D. (1995). Psychoeducation in First Episode Psychosis: A Therapeutic Process. *Psychiatry*, **58**, 313–28.

McGorry, P. D., & McConville, S. B. (1999). Insight in Psychosis: An Elusive Target. *Comprehensive Psychiatry*, **40** (2), 131–42.

McManamy, J. (2007). *McMan's Depression and Bipolar Report*, **9** (19), 1–8.

Merikangas, K. R., Akiskal H. S., Angst, J., et al. (2007). Lifetime and 12-Month Prevalence of Bipolar Spectrum Disorder in the National Comorbidity Survey Replication. *Archives of General Psychiatry*, **64** (5), 543–52.

Mester, R., Toren, P., Mizrachi, I., et al. (1995). Caffeine Withdrawal Increases Lithium Blood Levels. *Biological Psychiatry*, **37**, 348–50.

Meyer, B., Pilkonis, P. A., Krupnick, J. L., et al. (2002). Treatment Expectancies, Patient Alliance, and Outcome: Further Analyses from the National Institute of Mental Health Treatment of Depression Collaborative Research Program. *Journal of Consulting and Clinical Psychology*, **70** (4), 1051–5.

Meyer, T. D., & Maier, S. (2006). Is There Evidence for Social Rhythm Instability in People at Risk for Affective Disorders? *Psychiatry Research*, **141**, 103–14.

Miklowitz, D. J. (2002). *The Bipolar Disorder Survival Guide*. New York: Guilford Press.

Miklowitz, D. J. (2008). *Bipolar Disorder: A Family-Focused Treatment Approach*, 2nd edn. New York: Guilford Press.

Miklowitz, D. J., & Goldstein, M. J. (1997). *Bipolar Disorder: A Family-Focused Treatment Approach*. New York: Guilford Press.

Miklowitz, D. J., Goldstein, M. J., & Nuechterlein, K. H. (1995). Verbal Interactions in the Families of Schizophrenic and Bipolar Affective Patients. *Journal of Abnormal Psychology*, **104** (2), 268–76.

Miklowitz, D. J., Goldstein, M. J., Nuechterlein, K. H., Snyder, K. S., & Mintz, J. (1988). Family Factors and the Course of Bipolar Affective Disorder. *Archives of General Psychiatry*, **45** (3), 225–31.

Miklowitz, D. J., & Hooley, J. M. (1998). Developing Family Psychoeducational Treatments for Patients with Bipolar and Other Severe Psychiatric Disorders. A Pathway from Basic Research to Clinical Trials. *Journal of Marital and Family Therapy*, **24** (4), 419–35.

Miklowitz, D. J., Otto, M. W., Frank, E., et al. (2007a). Psychosocial Treatments for Bipolar Depression: A 1-Year Randomized Trial from the Systematic Treatment Enhancement Program. *Archives of General Psychiatry*, **64** (4), 419–27.

Miklowitz, D. J., Otto, M. W., Frank, E., et al. (2007b). Intensive Psychosocial Intervention Enhances Functioning in Patients with Bipolar Depression: Results from a 9-Month Randomized Controlled Trial. *American Journal of Psychiatry*. **164** (9), 1340–7.

Miller, W. R., & Rollnick, S. (2002). *Motivational Interviewing: Preparing People for Change*, 2nd edn. New York: Guilford Press.

Mintz, A. R., Dobson, K. S., & Romney, D. M. (2003). Insight in Schizophrenia: A Meta Analysis. *Schizophrenia Research*, **61**, 75–88.

Mitchell, P. B., & Malhi, G. S. (2004). Bipolar Depression: Phenomenological Overview and Clinical Characteristics. *Bipolar Disorders*, **6** (6), 530–9.

Molnar, G., Feeney, M. G., & Fava, G. A. (1988). Duration and Symptoms of Bipolar Prodromes. *American Journal of Psychiatry*, **145** (12), 1576–8.

Monk, T. H., Flaherty, J. F., Frank, E., Hoskinson, K., & Kupfer, D. J. (1990). The Social Rhythm Metric: An Instrument to Quantify the Daily Rhythms of Life. *Journal of Nervous and Mental Disease*, **178**, 120–6.

Mooney, K. A., & Padesky, C. A. (2000). Applying Client Creativity to Recurrent Problems: Constructing Possibilities and Tolerating Doubt. *Journal of Cognitive Psychotherapy: An International Quarterly*, **14** (2), 149–61.

Morgenson, G. (1996). Escaping to the Angels: A Note on the Passing of the Manic Defence. *Journal of Analytic Psychology*, **41**, 77–80.

Morriss, R. (2002). Clinical Importance of Inter-Episode Symptoms in Patients with Bipolar Affective Disorder. *Journal of Affective Disorders*, **72** (Suppl. 1), S3–13.

Morriss, R. K., Faizal, M. A., Jones, A. P., et al. (2007). Interventions for Helping People Recognise Early Signs of Recurrence in Bipolar Disorder. *Cochrane Database of Systematic Reviews*, (1), CD004854.

Morselli, P. L., & Elgie, R. (2003). GAMIAN-Europe/BEAM Survey I – Global Analysis of a Patient Questionnaire Circulated to 3450 Members of 12 European Advocacy Groups Operating in the Field of Mood Disorders. *Bipolar Disorders*, **5**, 265–78.

Mueser, K. T., & Glynn, S. M. (1999). *Behavioral Family Therapy for Psychiatric Disorders*, 2nd edn. Oakland, CA: New Harbinger Publications.

Muller-Oerlinghausen, B., Wolf, T., Ahrens, B., et al. (1996). Mortality of Patients Who Dropped Out from Regular Lithium Prophylaxis. *Acta Psychiatrica Scandinavica*, **94**, (5), 344–7.

Murray, C. J. L., & Lopez, A. D. (1996). *The Global Burden of Disease: A Comprehensive Assessment of Mortality and Disability from Diseases, Injuries and Risk Factors in 1990 and Projected to 2020*. Boston: Harvard University Press.

National Institute for Health and Clinical Excellence (NICE) (2006). *The Management of Bipolar Disorder in Adults, Children and Adolescents, in Primary and Secondary Care*. London: NICE.

Neale, J. M. (1988). Defensive Function of Manic Episodes. In Oltmans, T. F., & Maher, B. A., eds., *Delusional Beliefs*. New York: John Wiley & Sons, Ltd., 138–56.

Newman, C., Leahy, R. L., Beck, A. T., Reilly-Harrington, N. A., & Gyulai, L. (2002). *Bipolar Disorder: A Cognitive Approach*. Washington: American Psychological Association.

Ng, F., Dodd, S., & Berk, M. (2007). The Effects of Physical Activity in the Acute Treatment of Bipolar Disorder: A Pilot Study. *Journal of Affective Disorders*, **101** (1–3), 259–62.

Norman, R., & Malla, A. (1994). Prodromal Symptoms in Schizophrenia. *British Journal of Psychiatry*, **164**, 487–93.

O'Hanlon, W. H., & Weiner-Davis, M. (1989). *In Search of Solutions: A New Direction in Psychotherapy*. New York: Norton.

Olivier, D., Lubman, D. I., & Fraser, R. (2007). Tobacco Smoking within Psychiatric Inpatient Settings: A Biopsychosocial Perspective. *Australian and New Zealand Journal of Psychiatry*, **41** (7), 572–80.

Orlinsky, D. E., & Howard, K. I. (1986). The Psychological Interior of Psychotherapy: Explorations with the Therapy Session Reports. In Greenberg, L. S., & Pinsoff, W. M., eds., *The Psychotherapeutic Process: A Research Handbook*. New York: Guilford Press.

Otto, M. W., Perlman, C. A., Wernicke, R., et al. (2004). Posttraumatic Stress Disorder in Patients with Bipolar Disorder: A Review of Prevalence, Correlates and Treatment Strategies. *Bipolar Disorders*, **6** (6), 470–9.

Overholser, J. C. (1993). Elements of the Socratic Method: I. Systematic Questioning. *Psychotherapy*, **30** (1), 67–74.

Padesky, C. A. (1993). *Socratic Questioning: Changing Minds or Guiding Discovery?* Keynote address delivered at the European Congress of Behavioural and Cognitive Therapies, London.

Padesky, C. A. (1994). Schema Change Processes in Cognitive Therapy. *Clinical Psychology and Psychotherapy*, **1** (5), 267–78.

Padesky, C. A. (2000). *Transforming Personality: In-Depth Training in Cognitive Therapy of Personality Disorders*. Workshop presented in London, England.

Padesky, C. A., & Mooney, K. A. (1990). Clinical Tip: Presenting the Cognitive Model to Clients. *International Cognitive Therapy Newsletter*, **6**, 13–14.

Pallanti, S., Quercioli, L., Pazzagli, A., et al. (1999). Awareness of Illness and Subjective Experience of Cognitive Complaints in Patients with Bipolar I and Bipolar II Disorder. *American Journal of Psychiatry*, **156** (7), 1094–6.

Pardoen, D., Bauwens, F., Tracy, A., Martin, F., & Mendlewicz, J. (1993). Self-Esteem in Recovered Bipolar and Unipolar Outpatients. *British Journal of Psychiatry*, **163**, 755–62.

Pasco, J. A., Williams, L. J., Jacka, F. N., et al. (2008). Tobacco Smoking as a Risk Factor for Major Depressive Disorder: Population-based Study. *British Journal of Psychiatry*, **193** (4), 322–6.

Pavuluri, M. N., Graczyk, P. A., Henry, D. B., et al. (2004). Child and Family-Focused Cognitive Behavioural Therapy for Pediatric Bipolar Disorder: Development and Preliminary Results. *Journal of the American Academy of Child and Adolescent Psychiatry*, **43**, 528–37.

Paykel, E. S., Abbott, R., Morriss, R., Hayhurst, H., & Scott, J. (2006). Sub-syndromal and Syndromal Symptoms in the Longitudinal Course of Bipolar Disorder. *British Journal of Psychiatry*, **189**, 118–23.

Peet, M., & Harvey, N. S. (1991). Lithium Maintenance 1. A Standard Education Programme for Patients. *British Journal of Psychiatry*, **158**, 197–200.

Peeters, F., Wessel, I., Merckelbach, H., & Boon-Vermeeren, M. (2002). Autobiographical Memory Specificity and the Course of Major Depressive Disorder. *Comprehensive Psychiatry*, **43** (5), 344–50.

Pekkala, E., & Merinder, L. (2002). Psychoeducation for Schizophrenia (Review). *Cochrane Database of Systematic Reviews*, (2), CD002831.

Pekkarinen, P., Terwilliger, J., Bredbacka, P. E., Lonnqvist J., & Peltonen L. (1995). Evidence of a Predisposing Locus to Bipolar Disorder on Xq24–q27.1 in an Extended Finnish Pedigree. *Genome Research*, **5** (2), 105–15.

Penedo, F. J., & Dahn, J. R. (2005). Exercise and Well-Being: A Review of Mental and Physical Health Benefits Associated with Physical Activity. *Current Opinion in Psychiatry*, **18**, 189–93.

Perlick, D. A., Rosenheck, R. A., Clarkin, J. F., et al. (2001). Adverse Effects of Perceived Stigma on Social Adaptation of Persons Diagnosed with Bipolar Affective Disorder. *Psychiatric Services*, **52** (12), 1627–32.

Perlis, R. H., Miyahara, S., Marangell, L. B., et al. (2004). Long-Term Implications of Early Onset in Bipolar Disorder: Data From the First 1000 Participants in the Systematic Treatment Enhancement Program for Bipolar Disorder (STEP-BD). *Biological Psychiatry*, **55** (9), 875–81.

Perry, A., Tarrier, N., & Morriss, R. (1995). Identification of Prodromal Signs and Symptoms and Early Intervention in Manic Depressive Patients: A Case Example. *Behavioural and Cognitive Psychotherapy*, **23**, 399–409.

Perry, A., Tarrier, N., Morriss, R., McCarthy, E., & Limb, K. (1999). Randomised Controlled Trial of Efficacy of Teaching Patients with Bipolar Disorder to Identify Early Symptoms of Relapse and Obtain Treatment. *British Medical Journal*, **318**, 139–53.

Persons, J. B. (2006). Case Formulation-Driven Psychotherapy. *Clinical Psychology: Science and Practice*, **13**, 167–70.

Phelps, J., Angst, J., Katzow, J., & Sadler, J. (2008). Validity and Utility of Bipolar Spectrum Models. *Bipolar Disorders*, **10** (1), 179–93.

Pini, S., Cassano, G. B., Dell'Osso, L., & Amador, X. F. (2001). Insight into Illness in Schizophrenia, Schizoaffective Disorder, and Mood Disorders with Psychotic Features. *American Journal of Psychiatry*, **158** (1), 122–5.

Pope, M., Dudley, R., & Scott, J. (2007). Determinants of Social Functioning in Bipolar Disorder. *Bipolar Disorders*, **9**, 38–44.

Pope, M., & Scott, J. (2003). Do Clinicians Understand Why Individuals Stop Taking Lithium? *Journal of Affective Disorders*, **74** (3), 287–91.

Post, R. M. (1992). Transduction of Psychological Stress into the Neurobiology of Recurrent Affective Disorder. *American Journal of Psychiatry*, **149**, 999–1010.

Post, R. M., Leverich, G. S., Xing, G., & Weiss, S. R. B. (2001). Developmental Vulnerabilities to the Onset and Course of Bipolar Disorder. *Development & Psychopathology*, **13** (3), 581–98.

Post, R. M., Rubinow, D. R., & Ballenger, J. C. (1986). Conditioning and Sensitisation in the Longitudinal Course of Affective Illness. *British Journal of Psychiatry*, **149**, 191–201.

Potash, J. B., Kane, H. S., Chiu, Y. F., et al. (2000). Attempted Suicide and Alcoholism in Bipolar Disorder: Clinical and Familial Relationships. *American Journal of Psychiatry*, **157** (12), 2048–50.

Power, M. J. (2005). Psychological Approaches to Bipolar Disorders: A Theoretical Critique. *Clinical Psychology Review*, **25**, 1101–22.

Priebe, S., & Gruyters, T. (1995). The Importance of the First Three Days: Predictors of Treatment Outcome in Depressed Inpatients. *British Journal of Clinical Psychology*, **34** (2), 229–36.

Prien, R. F., Kupfer, D. J., Mansky, P. A., et al. (1984). Drug Therapy in the Prevention of Recurrences in Unipolar and Bipolar Affective Disorders. *Archives of General Psychiatry*, **41**, 1096–104.

Prien, R. F., & Potter, W. Z. (1990). NIMH Workshop Report on Treatment of Bipolar Disorder. *Psychopharmacology Bulletin*, **26** (4), 409–27.

Prochaska, J. O., & DiClemente, C. C. (1986). Towards a Comprehensive Model of Change. In Miller, W. R., & Heather, N., eds., *Treating Addictive Behaviors: Processes of Change*. Homewood, Illinois: Dow Jones/Irwin.

Ramirez-Basco, M., & Rush, A. J. (1996). *Cognitive Behavioural Therapy for Bipolar Disorder*. New York: Guilford Press.

Ramirez-Basco, M., & Rush, A. J. (2007). *Cognitive Behavioural Therapy for Bipolar Disorder*, 2nd edn. New York: Guilford Press.

Rees, C. S., McEvoy, P., & Nathan, P. R. (2005). Relationship Between Homework Completion and Outcome in Cognitive Behaviour Therapy. *Cognitive Behaviour Therapy*, **34** (4), 242–7.

Regier, D. A., Farmer, M. E., Rae, D. S., et al. (1990). Comorbidity of Mental Disorders with Alcohol and Other Drug Abuse. Results from the Epidemiologic Catchment Area (ECA) Study. *Journal of the American Medical Association*, **264** (19), 2511–18.

Riedel, B. W., Lichstein, K. L., Peterson, B. A., et al. (1998). A Comparison of the Efficacy of Stimulus Control for Medicated and Nonmedicated Insomniacs. *Behavior Modification*, **22** (1), 3–28.

Rogers, C. R. (1976). *Client Centred Therapy*. London: Constable & Robinson.

Royal Australian and New Zealand College of Psychiatrists (2004). Australian and New Zealand Clinical Practice Guidelines for Treatment of Bipolar Disorder. *Australian and New Zealand Journal of Psychiatry*, **38**, 280–305.

Roy-Byrne, P., Post, R. M., Uhde, T. W., Porcu, T., & Davis, D. (1985). The Longitudinal Course of Recurrent Affective Illness: Life Chart Data from Research Patients at the NIMH. *Acta Psychiatrica Scandinavica, Supplementum*, **317**, 1–34.

Rush, A. J. (1988). Cognitive Approaches to Adherence. In Frances, A., & Hales, R., eds., *Review of Psychiatry* (Vol 8). Washington, DC: American Psychiatric Association, 627–42.

Russell, S. J., & Browne, J. L. (2005). Staying Well with Bipolar Disorder. *Australian and New Zealand Journal of Psychiatry*, **39**, 187–93.

Ryle, A., & Kerr, I. (2002). *Introducing Cognitive Analytic Therapy: Principles and Practice*. West Sussex: John Wiley & Sons, Ltd.

Sachs, G. (2003). Unmet Needs in Bipolar Disorder. *Journal of Clinical Psychopharmacology*, **23** (Suppl. 1), S2–8.

Sackeim, H. A. (1998). The Meaning of Insight. In Amador, X. F., & Davids, A. S., eds., *Insight and Psychosis*. New York: Oxford University Press.

Salloum, I. M., & Thase, M. E. (2000). Impact of Substance Use on the Course and Treatment of Bipolar Disorder. *Bipolar Disorders*, **2**, 269–80.

Satterfield, J. M. (1999). Adjunctive Cognitive Behavioral Therapy for Rapid Cycling Bipolar Disorder: An Empirical Case Study. *Psychiatry*, **62** (4), 357–69.

Saunders, J. B., Aasland, O. G., Babor, T. F., de le Fuente, J. R., & Grant, M. (1993). Development of the Alcohol Use Disorders Identification Test (AUDIT). WHO Collaborative Project on Early Detection of Persons with Harmful Alcohol Consumption. *Addiction*, **88**, 791–804.

Schwannauer, M. (2003). Cognitive Behavioural Therapy for Bipolar Affective Disorder. In Power, M., ed., *A Handbook of Science and Practice: Mood Disorders*. West Sussex: John Wiley & Sons, Ltd.

Schwartz, B., & Flowers, J. V. (2006). *How to Fail as a Therapist*. California: Impact Publishers.

Scott, J. (1995). Psychotherapy for Bipolar Disorder. *British Journal of Psychiatry*, **167** (5), 581–8.

Scott, J. (1996). Cognitive Therapy for Clients with Bipolar Disorder. *Cognitive and Behavioural Practice*, **3**, 29–51.

Scott, J. (2001). *Overcoming Mood Swings*. London: Robinson.

Scott, J. (2003). Cognitive Theory and Therapy of Bipolar Disorders. In Reinecke, M., & Clarke, D. A., eds., *Cognitive Therapy Across the Life Span*. Cambridge: Cambridge University Press.

Scott, J. (2008). Cognitive Therapy for Severe Mental Disorders: Back to the Future? *British Journal of Psychiatry*, **192**, 401–3.

Scott, J., & Colom, F. (2005). Psychological Treatments for Bipolar Disorders. *Psychiatric Clinics of North America*, **28** (2), 371–84.

Scott, J., & Colom, F. (2008). Gaps and Limitations of Psychological Interventions for Bipolar Disorders. *Psychotherapy and Psychosomatics*, **77** (1), 4–11.

Scott, J., Garland, A., & Moorhead, S. (2001). A Pilot Study of Cognitive Therapy in Bipolar Disorders. *Psychological Medicine*, **31** (3), 459–67.

Scott, J., & Gutierrez, M. J. (2004). The Current Status of Psychological Treatments in Bipolar Disorders: A Systematic Review of Relapse Prevention. *Bipolar Disorders*, **6**, 498–503.

Scott, J., Paykel, E., Morriss, R., et al. (2006). Cognitive-Behavioural Therapy for Severe and Recurrent Bipolar Disorders: Randomised Controlled Trial. *British Journal of Psychiatry*, **188**, 313–20.

Scott, J., & Pope, M. (2002). Non-Adherence with Mood Stabilisers: Prevalence and Predictors. *Journal of Clinical Psychology*, **63**, 384–90.

Scott, J., Stanton, B., Garland, A., & Ferrier, I. N. (2000). Cognitive Vulnerability in Patients with Bipolar Disorder. *Psychological Medicine*, **30**, 467–72.

Scott, J., & Tacchi, M. J. (2002). A Pilot Study of Concordance Therapy for Individuals with Bipolar Disorders who are Non-Adherent with Lithium Prophylaxis. *Bipolar Disorders*, **4**, 386–92.

Seiffgre-Krenke, I. (2000). Causal Links Between Stressful Events, Coping Style, and Adolescent Symptomatology. *Journal of Adolescence*, **23**, 675–91.

Shakespeare, W. (1999). *The Complete Works*. Hertfordshire: Wordsworth Editions Ltd.

Silverstone, T., McPherson, H., Hunt, N., & Romans, S. (1998). How Effective is Lithium in the Prevention of Relapse in Bipolar Disorder? A Prospective Naturalistic Follow-Up Study. *Australian and New Zealand Journal of Psychiatry*, **32**, 61–6.

Simon, N. M., Otto, M. W., Wisniewski, S. R., et al. (2004). Anxiety Disorder Comorbidity in Bipolar Disorder Patients: Data from the First 500 Participants in the Systematic Treatment Enhancement Program for Bipolar Disorder (STEP-BD). *American Journal of Psychiatry*, **161** (12), 2222–9.

Simoneau, T. L., Miklowitz, D. J., & Saleem, R. (1998). Expressed Emotion and Interactional Patterns in the Families of Bipolar Patients. *Journal of Abnormal Psychology*, **107** (3), 497–507.

Simpson, J. B. (1988). *Simpson's Contemporary Quotations*. Massachusetts: Houghton Mifflin Company.

Sklar, P., Smoller, J. W., Fan, J., et al. (2008). Whole-Genome Association Study of Bipolar Disorder. *Molecular Psychiatry*, **13** (6), 558–69.

Smith, J. A., & Tarrier, N. (1992). Prodromal Symptoms in Manic Depressive Psychosis. *Social Psychiatry and Psychiatric Epidemiology*, **27**, 245–8.

Steinberg, D. (1987). *Basic Adolescent Psychiatry*. Oxford: Blackwell Scientific Publications.

Stepanski, E. J., & Wyatt, J. K. (2003). Use of Sleep Hygiene in the Treatment of Insomnia. *Sleep Medicine Reviews*, **7** (3), 215–25.

Strakowski, S. M., DelBello, M. P., Zimmerman, M. E., et al. (2002). Ventricular and Periventricular Structural Volumes in First- Versus Multiple-Episode Bipolar Disorder. *American Journal of Psychiatry*, **159** (11), 1841–7.

Strakowski, S. M., Peck, P. E., McElroy, S. L., et al. (1998). Twelve Month Outcome after a First Hospitalization for Affective Psychosis. *Archives of General Psychiatry*, **55** (1), 49–55.

Strakowski, S. M., Williams, J. R., Fleck, D. E., & Delbello, M. P. (2000). Eight Month Functional Outcome from Mania following a First Psychiatric Hospitalization. *Journal of Psychiatric Research*, **34** (3), 193–200.

Strober, M., Morrell, W., Lampert, C., & Burroughs, J. (1990). Relapse Following Discontinuation of Lithium Maintenance Therapy in Adolescents with Bipolar I Illness: A Naturalistic Study. *American Journal of Psychiatry*, **147** (4), 457–61.

Sullivan, M. F., Skovholt, T. M., & Jennings, L. (2005). Master Therapists' Construction of the Therapy Relationship. *Journal of Mental Health Counseling*, **27** (1), 48–70.

Swann, A. C., Bowden, C. L., Calabrese, J. R., Dilsaver, S. C., & Morris, D. D. (1999). Differential Effect of Number of Previous Episodes of Affective Disorder on Response to Lithium or Divalproex in Acute Mania. *American Journal of Psychiatry*, **156** (8), 1264–6.

Swartz, H. A., & Frank, E. (2001). Psychotherapy for Bipolar Depression: A Phase-Specific Treatment Strategy. *Bipolar Disorders*, **3**, 11–22.

Swayze, V. W., Andreasen, N. C., Alliger, R. J., Ehrhardt, J. C., & Yuh, W. T. (1990). Structural Brain Abnormalities in Bipolar Affective Disorder. *Archives of General Psychiatry*, **47** (11), 1054–9.

Swofford, C., Kasckow, D., Scheller-Gilkey, G., & Inderbitzin, L. B. (1996). Substance Use: A Powerful Predictor of Relapse in Schizophrenia. *Schizophrenia Research*, **20** (1–2), 145–51.

Tacchi, M. J., & Scott, J. (2005). *Improving Adherence in Schizophrenia and Bipolar Disorders*. West Sussex: John Wiley & Sons, Ltd.

Tait, A., McNay, L., Gumley, A., & O'Grady, M. (2002). The Development and Implementation of an Individualised Early Signs Monitoring System in the Prediction of Relapse in Schizophrenia. *Journal of Mental Health*, **11** (2), 141–53.

Targum, S. D., Dibble, E. D., Davenport, Y. B., & Gershon, E. S. (1981). The Family Attitude Scale: Patients' and Spouses' View of Bipolar Illness. *Archives of General Psychiatry*, **38**, 562–8.

Taylor, H. (1999). Explosive Growth of a New Breed of "Cyberchondriacs." *The Harris Poll* #11, Feb 17.

Teasdale, J. D., & Barnard, P. J. (1993). *Affect, Cognition and Change: Re-Modeling Depressive Thought*. East Sussex: Lawrence Erlbaum Associates.

Terr, L. C., Deeney, J. M., Drell, M., et al. (2006). Playful "Moments" in Psychotherapy. *Journal of the American Academy of Child and Adolescent Psychiatry*, **45** (5), 604–13.

Teyber, E., & McClure, F. (2000). Therapist Variables. In Snyder, C. R., & Ingram, R. E., eds., *Handbook of Psychological Change*. New York: John Wiley & Sons, Ltd.

Thomas, J., Knowles, R., Tai, S., & Bentall, R. P. (2007). Response Styles to Depressed Mood in Bipolar Affective Disorder. *Journal of Affective Disorders*, **100**, 249–52.

Thompson, K. N., Phillips, L. J., Komesaroff, P., et al. (2007). Stress and HPA-Axis Functioning in Young People at Ultra High Risk for Psychosis. *Journal of Psychiatric Research*, **41** (7), 561–9.

Timbremont, B., & Braet, C. (2004). Cognitive Vulnerability in Remitted Depressed Children and Adolescents. *Behaviour Research and Therapy*, **42**, 423–37.

Tohen, M., Hennen, J., Zarate, C. M., et al. (2000). Two Year Syndromal and Functional Recovery in 219 Cases of First Episode Major Affective Disorder with Psychotic Features. *American Journal of Psychiatry*, **157** (2), 220–8.

Tohen, M., Waternaux, C. M., & Tsuang, M. T. (1990). Outcome in Mania: A 4-Year Prospective Follow-Up of 75 Patients Utilizing Survival Analysis. *Archives of General Psychiatry*, **47** (12), 1106–11.

Torrey, E. F., & Knable, M. B. (2002). *Surviving Manic Depression*. New York: Basic Books.

Turner, de S., & Cox, H. (2004). Facilitating Post Traumatic Growth. *Health and Quality of Life Outcomes*, **2**, 34.

Wallace, C. J., & Tauber, R. (2004). Supplementing Supported Employment with Workplace Skills Training. *Psychiatric Services*, **55** (5), 513–15.

Wallace, C. J., Tauber, R., & Wilde, J. (1999). Teaching Fundamental Workplace Skills to Persons with Serious Mental Illness. *Psychiatric Services*, **50** (9), 1147–53.

Ward, J. L., Conus, P. O., Allen, N., et al. (2003). The Initial Manic Prodrome: Implications for Early Detection & Intervention. *Schizophrenia Research*, **60** (1), 29–30.

Waters, B., & Calleia, S. (1983). The Effect of Juvenile-Onset Manic-Depressive Disorder on the Developmental Tasks of Adolescence. *American Journal of Psychotherapy*, **37** (2), 182–9.

Wehr, T. A., Sack, D. A., & Rosenthal, N. E. (1987). Sleep Reduction as the Final Common Pathway in the Genesis of Mania. *American Journal of Psychiatry*, **144**, 201–4.

Weinberger, J., & Eig, A. (1999). Expectancies: The Ignored Common Factor in Psychotherapy. In Kirsch, I., ed., *How Expectancies Shape Experience*. Washington DC: American Psychological Association, 357–82.

Weingartner, H., Miller, H., & Murphy, D. L. (1977). Mood State Dependent Retrieval of Verbal Associations. *Journal of Abnormal Psychology*, **86**, 276–84.

Weissman, A. N., & Beck, A. T. (1978). *Development and Validation of the Dysfunctional Attitudes Scale*. Paper presented at the annual meeting of the Association for the Advancement of Behavior Therapy, Chicago.

Wendel, J. S., & Miklowitz, D. J. (1997). *Attribution and Expressed Emotion in the Relatives of Patients with Bipolar Disorder*. Poster presented at the 31st Annual Conference of the Association for the Advancement of Behavior Therapy, Miami Beach, Florida.

Wender, R. C. (1996). Humor in Medicine. *Primary Care*, **23**, 141–54.

Wessel, I., Meeren, M., Peeters, F., Arntz, A., & Merckelbach, H. (2001). Correlates of Autobiographical Memory Specificity: The Role of Depression, Anxiety and Childhood Trauma. *Behaviour Research and Therapy*, **39**, 409–21.

White, R. G., McCleery, M., Gumley, A. I., & Mulholland, C. (2007). Hopelessness in Schizophrenia: The Impact of Symptoms and Beliefs about Illness. *Journal of Nervous and Mental Disease*, **195** (12), 968–75.

Williams, C. C., & Collins, A. (2002). Factors Associated with Insight Among Outpatients with Serious Mental Illness. *Psychiatric Services*, **53** (1), 96–8.

Winters, K. C., & Neale, J. M. (1985). Mania and Low Self-Esteem. *Journal of Abnormal Psychology*, **94** (3), 282–90.

Woodward, C., & Joseph, S. (2003). Positive Change and Post-Traumatic Growth in People who have Experienced Childhood Abuse: Understanding Vehicles of Change. *Psychology & Psychotherapy: Theory, Research and Practice*, **76**, 267–83.

World Health Organization ASSIST Working Group (2002). The Alcohol, Smoking and Substance Involvement Screening Test (ASSIST): Development, Reliability and Feasibility. *Addiction*, **97**, 1183–94.

Yalom, I. D. (1999). *Momma and the Meaning of Life: Tales of Psychotherapy*. London: Piatkus.

Yalom, I. D. (2002). *The Gift of Therapy: Reflections on Being a Therapist*. London: Piatkus.

Yen, C. F., Chen, C. S., Ko, C. H., et al. (2005). Relationships Between Insight and Medication Adherence in Outpatients with Schizophrenia and Bipolar Disorder: Prospective Study. *Psychiatry and Clinical Neurosciences*, **59** (4), 403–9.

Yen, C. F., Chen, C. S., Yeh, M. L., et al. (2002). Comparison of Insight in Patients with Schizophrenia and Bipolar Disorder in Remission. *Journal of Nervous and Mental Disease*, **190** (12), 847–9.

Young, J. E., & Brown, G. (2005). *Young Schema Questionnaire*. New York: Cognitive Therapy Centre of New York.

Young, J. E., & Klosko, J. S. (1993). *Reinventing Your Life*. New York: Penguin Putnam Inc.

Young, J. E., Klosko, J. S., & Weishaar, M. (2003). *Schema Therapy: A Practitioner's Guide*. New York: Guilford Press.

Young, R. C., Biggs, J. T., Ziegler, V. E., & Meyer, D. A. (1978). A Rating Scale for Mania: Reliability, Validity, and Sensitivity. *British Journal of Psychiatry*, **133**, 429–35.

Zaretsky, A. (2003). Targeted Psychosocial Interventions for Bipolar Disorder. *Bipolar Disorders*, **5** (Suppl. 2), 80–7.

Zaretsky, A. E., Segal, Z. V., & Gemar, M. (1999). Cognitive Therapy for Bipolar Depression: A Pilot Study. *Canadian Journal of Psychiatry*, **44** (5), 491–4.

Zimmerman, M., Chelminski, I., & Posternak, M. A. (2005). Generalizability of Antidepressant Efficacy Trials: Differences Between Depressed Psychiatric Outpatients Who Would or Would Not Qualify for an Efficacy Trial. *The American Journal of Psychiatry*, **162** (7), 1370–2.

Zis, A. P., Grof, P., Webster, M., & Goodwin, F. K. (1980). Prediction of Relapse in Recurrent Affective Disorder. *Psychopharmacology Bulletin*, **16** (1), 47–9.

Zubieta, J. K., Huguelet, P., Ohl, L. E., & Kroepe, R. A. (2000). High Vesicular Monoamine Transporter Binding in Asymptomatic Bipolar I Disorder. *American Journal of Psychiatry*, **157**, 1619–28.

Zubin, J., & Spring, B. (1977). Vulnerability – a New View on Schizophrenia. *Journal of Abnormal Psychology*, **86**, 103–26.

Index

Printed in the United States
By Bookmasters